the **yoga** year

celia**toler**

STOREY BOOKS

The mission of Storey Publishing is to serve our customers by publishing practical information that encourages personal independence in harmony with the environment.

United States edition published in 2001 by Storey Books,
210 MASS MoCA Way, North Adams, MA 01247

United Kingdom edition published in 2001 by MQ Publications Ltd,
12 The Ivories, 6–8 Northampton Street, London N1 2HY

Editor: Kate John, MQ Publications Ltd; Janet Lape, Storey Publishing
Editorial Director: Ljiljana Baird, MQ Publications Ltd; Deborah Balmuth, Storey Publishing
Art Direction: John Casey, MQ Publications Ltd; Meredith Maker, Storey Publishing
Illustrator: Penny Brown

Printed in China

Library of Congress Cataloging-in-Publication Data

Toler, Celia
The yoga year : a seasonal guide to asanas, breathing exercises, and inspiration / by Celia Toler.
p. cm.
ISBN 1-58017-426-4 (alk. Paper)
1. Yoga, Haoha. 2. Breathing exercises. 3. Inspiration. I. Title.

RA781.7 .T585 2001
613.7'046—dc21

2001041133

contents

introduction

Yoga is a wonderful form of exercise. It tones and strengthens the body by relaxing and releasing the tightness in muscles, creating flexibility. It also quiets and focuses the mind. The Yoga Year is a special book which presents a practical guide, through monthly routines, enabling you to start and develop your own yoga practice goals. The seasonal divisions of the routines are an aid to realizing these goals. Each month's ethos is followed by poses and concludes with breathing and relaxation techniques. Later, to maintain a rounded routine after the introduction of a new pose, familiar sequential poses are included. The routines are designed to be practiced in sequence since each month progresses and develops from the last.

If a new pose seems too difficult, another pose may act as a substitute. As you progress, look back at poses in previous months, which you can also include, develop, and make a routine that suits you. At the end of each month, The Story of Yoga unfolds with a wealth of background information on the history of this most ancient form of exercise.

To simplify things the structure of The Yoga Year book can be used exactly as it is and worked through month by month. At the same time, as it can take a whole year to complete, the seasonal sections show you where you can achieve results; for instance, in both the first and second quarters, the routines can be progressed more quickly than in the third and fourth.

Try to keep your sense of enjoyment and discovery at the forefront while approaching your practice sensibly: In yoga, you have a precious tool that will be useful in all of your life.

From a practical point of view, yoga is good for health. As it increases flexibility it also increases a feeling of well-being, which is harder to define but comes with diligent practice. Most importantly, its techniques of relaxation, both physically and mentally, help to counter stress from modern-day living, all of the year round.

The yoga within this book comes under the style referred to as Hatha yoga and has three principles:

❶ The use of gravity to make the base of the pose stable
❷ The lengthening of the spine from this stable base, and
❸ The use of the breath, which releases the spine so that it can lengthen.

These principles were developed by Vanda Scaravelli after studying with B.K.S. Iyengar and T.K.V. Desikachar. I, in turn, learnt these through studying with teachers who had studied with Vanda. To them, Chloe Fremantle, Mary Stewart, and Sophy Hoare, I extend a debt of gratitude and my thanks.

general caution

If you are in doubt about your health or ability to do yoga, always ask and take the advice of your doctor. A general rule is to avoid a build-up of pressure at any time in the face and neck when the head is lower than the heart, in any of the poses. If this occurs, come upright, check that you have been breathing properly, that you have not been pushing into a pose, re-read the instructions and, if it continues, seek advice. Breathing should never be labored or breathless. For those who are pregnant, it is better to seek the advice of a qualified teacher since the scope of this book does not include the necessary advice.

spring

beginnings

Welcome to the start of your yoga year. Yoga is for everyone and there are no beginners, for each person is already good at something. Like dormant seeds beneath the enfolding blanket of winter's earth, your potential is there. Your first task is to smile (yoga is not so serious), turn the page, and enjoy practicing the poses, letting your breath bring them alive. Follow the first three months' yoga routines to increase your flexibility and improve your health and well-being. Each month's routine is easy to follow, and, while you are getting used to daily yoga practice, feel free to alternate the first three months' routines: Simply try to do the full routine, whichever one you choose.

month 1

month 2

month 3

month 1

The focus of the first month is a sequence of yoga postures for standing and bending, to establish a firm, steady foundation for every pose that follows in the yoga year. The Sanskrit names for asanas, or yoga poses, often refer to natural phenomena, and the standing pose uses the image of a mountain to convey strength and stability. The program of postures ends with breathing techniques, including Ujjayi, the simplest form of deep breathing.

key postures:

tadasana (MOUNTAIN POSE)

namaste 1 (REVERSE PRAYER)

parsvottanasana (PYRAMID POSE)

uttanasana (STANDING FORWARD BEND)

balasana (CHILD POSE)

adho mukha svanasana (DOWNWARD FACING DOG)

pranayama (UJJAYI—SIMPLE BREATHING)

relaxation (SAVASANA—CORPSE POSE)

how to start

❶ Practice in a quiet, well-ventilated room. It helps if the surface is level, and it is best to work on a non-slip mat.

❷ Wear loose clothes: A T-shirt with leggings or shorts, for example. To keep warm, add a sweatshirt. Bare feet are safest, and allow for increased sensitivity.

❸ Keep a belt, tie, or webbed piece of cloth nearby to help with some of the stretches.

❹ Start yoga slowly, and, as a beginner, don't hold any of the poses for long. Allow your body to warm up before asking more of it.

❺ Perform exercises equally on both sides of the body: Most people are stronger on one side.

❻ Remain in poses only if comfortable. If you pull or force a pose, you may injure yourself. It is more important to discover how your body works than to achieve the pose.

standing and bending

When the human skeleton evolved from using four legs to being upright on two, standing became a balance in itself. Because of inertia, muscles are used to keep the body static. Motion has its own energy, and in order to trap this, or take it into a vertical posture, you must first be aware that movement does not cease when you stand still. Your muscles are also working to keep the body's internal systems functioning. They pump blood throughout the body, and contract and relax as the lungs are filled and emptied. Standing is not rigid, but a constant process of physical adjustment.

Gravity, the downward force, is also at work. You might be aware of this standing at a bus stop: Shifting weight from one leg to the other, trying to disperse the force of gravity, but to stand easily, your body must balance its different masses above each other, like a well-built tower. This is the logic of good posture. At the base of the tower are the feet: If they are firmly rooted, the body can align itself above them.

Similarly, gravity works in bending. As the upper body bends, it is subject to gravity and could make the body topple over if the hips, legs, and feet did not counteract its weight. The strength of the lower body enables the upper body to be fluid and flexible.

tadasana (MOUNTAIN POSE)

In Sanskrit, tada means "mountain" and asana is "pose." Tadasana is therefore a pose in which the body stands as firm and upright as a mountain, the feet rooted in the earth while the upper body lengthens upward to the sky.

To stand upright easily, align the three main masses of the body—the pelvis, chest, and head—one above the other. The spine, attached to these masses, keeps them in place and, by lengthening, brings them into alignment. Coordinate the movement of the spine with the out-breath.

❶ Start by letting your breath quiet to its own rhythm, breathing through your nose.

❷ Now, as you breathe out, exhale down the body and feel yourself straighten down to your feet and up to the crown of your head.

❸ As the in-breath comes, let it return up the body naturally. If this is a new sensation and you become breathless, return to your regular way of breathing before trying again.

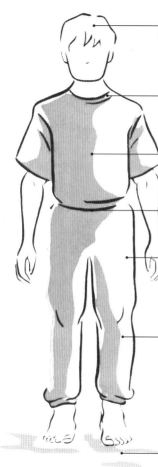

Keep the back of the neck long, with the head sitting easily on top, chin parallel to the ground. Let the space between the ears at the back of the head stay wide, the crown of the head grow upward.

Relax the shoulders, so they slope away from the ears, with the arms hanging like pendulums, wrists heavy, and hands relaxed.

With the out-breath, slide the front ribs down, making sure the chest does not jut out. Let the back ribs widen with the in-breath.

Breathe out into the back of the waist to help lengthen it.

Relax the buttocks and feel the hips wide and heavy. Keep the back of the pelvis straight, and drop the base of the spine toward the ground. Let the weight drop evenly down each leg.

Stand with knees straight, kneecaps relaxed, the back of the knees wide, but not overstretched. The muscles in the legs should be quiet.

Set the feet hip width apart, insides parallel to each other. Relax the toes, feeling the weight in the center of the heels and evenly balanced in each foot.

namaste 1 (REVERSE PRAYER)

To warm up for this exercise, stand and swing your arms gently. Exhale and take them above your head. Keep your shoulders down, with your arms dropped back into the shoulder sockets. On an out-breath, bring the arms down.

❶ Take the arms behind the body, and place the palms of the hands together with fingers pointing downward.

❷ Turn the fingers in toward the spine and slide them up, palms together. If you cannot turn the hands inward, hold your lower arms behind you, working each hand toward the opposite elbow.

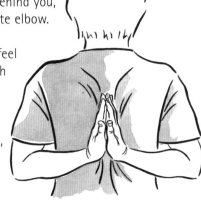

❸ Relax the shoulders so the elbows feel heavy. Breathe out, and feel the breath behind your hands, moving down the backbone.

❹ Hold only as long as is comfortable, then release the hands and shake the wrists gently.

forward bends

Both the asanas that follow begin from a strong base in the legs and feet, the feet starting as in Tadasana *(see pages 14–15)*. With the exhalation, the backbone lengthens forward and down.

When practicing forward bends, flex at the hips rather than at the waist to protect the lower back. The lumbar vertebrae lengthen with the exhalation, which helps the hips become more mobile and prevents strain. Always move on the out-breath.

Vary the length of time you hold these poses according to how comfortable your body is. Don't hold them for long if you feel uncomfortable: Five cycles of breath is sufficient to begin with.

If desired, both poses can be performed with the hands in Reverse Prayer I *(see page 18)*, or with arms folded loosely behind you. You won't be able to bend so far forward, but your back will remain straighter.

If you suffer from back pain, practice both forward bends toward a chair, to allow your legs and hips, not your back, to support the movement. Rest your wrists on the back of the chair rather than holding it with your hands. Place the chair far enough away that there is enough room for the upper body and arms to stretch out but that your heels stay flat on the ground in the pose. The back lengthens and relaxes.

parsvottanasana

(PYRAMID POSE)

Stand with feet parallel, hip-width apart; take the weight on your left leg. Move the right leg forward. On the exhalation, bend forward. Breathe for a few cycles. Come upright on an exhalation, using the back heel as an anchor, and uncurling from the base of the spine. Repeat the pose on your left leg.

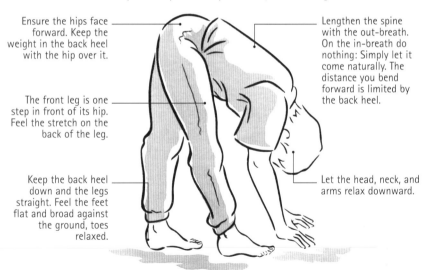

Ensure the hips face forward. Keep the weight in the back heel with the hip over it.

The front leg is one step in front of its hip. Feel the stretch on the back of the leg.

Keep the back heel down and the legs straight. Feel the feet flat and broad against the ground, toes relaxed.

Lengthen the spine with the out-breath. On the in-breath do nothing: Simply let it come naturally. The distance you bend forward is limited by the back heel.

Let the head, neck, and arms relax downward.

uttanasana (STANDING FORWARD BEND)

Stand and fold your arms loosely in front of you. Exhale and bend forward from the hips. The weight of your arms takes you down. Breathe for a few cycles. Return upright on an exhalation, tail in and lower back rounded.

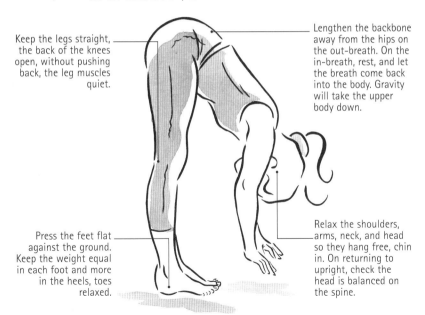

Keep the legs straight, the back of the knees open, without pushing back, the leg muscles quiet.

Lengthen the backbone away from the hips on the out-breath. On the in-breath, rest, and let the breath come back into the body. Gravity will take the upper body down.

Press the feet flat against the ground. Keep the weight equal in each foot and more in the heels, toes relaxed.

Relax the shoulders, arms, neck, and head so they hang free, chin in. On returning to upright, check the head is balanced on the spine.

balasana (CHILD POSE)

A stable pose, Child Pose is excellent for easing the lower
back, as it lengthens the spine, rounds out the inner curve
of the lower back, and widens the back of the pelvis.

  Body proportions can make Child Pose difficult, but it's
worth persevering for its ultimate restfulness. Try
stretching out to a chair, resting your head on your folded
arms on the seat—this lovely stretch in itself undoes knots
in the spine. Place cushions behind the knees and under
the thighs to ease stiffer hips. A rolled blanket, placed
under the ankles and the top of the feet, also helps.

❶ Kneel forward, placing the head on the arms. If this is
comfortable, take the arms apart and rest the forehead on
the floor. Then take the arms behind, resting them on the
ground, palms up.

❸ Exhale toward the back of the waist, and relax the hips.
As the in-breath comes, feel the back ribs widening. Stay
in the pose, breathing, as long as is comfortable.

This relaxing pose is very useful between other poses and good preparation for Downward Facing Dog *(see pages 22-23)*.

With the exhalation, lengthen the lower back and broaden the pelvis. Let the in-breath widen the back ribs.

Rest the forehead on the ground, with neck and shoulders relaxed.

Keep the knees together and drop the pelvis toward the heels.

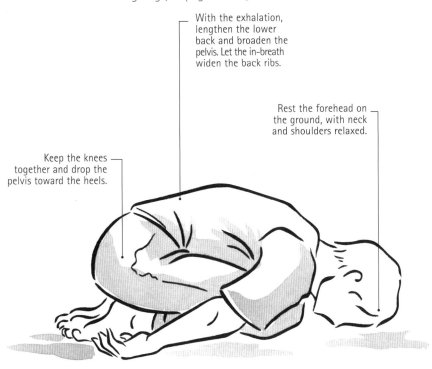

adho mukha svanasana

(DOWNWARD FACING DOG)

An invigorating asana and one which is best practiced using a non-slip mat, this resembles a dog stretching after lying down. The hands and feet are the roots of the pose, while the spine lengthens between them. It is excellent for easing a stiff neck, and for releasing the shoulders, which relax their weight down through the arms to the hands. It also gives the hips a good stretch. In this pose, tight hamstrings may keep the back of the legs tight and the heels up. The hamstrings need to be released, but avoid straining. Focus instead on lengthening the spine back to the hips, and on the heaviness in the roots, your hands and feet.

❶ From Child Pose *(see pages 20-21)*, lengthen the arms in front of you. Come up onto hands and knees, shoulders over hands and back straight. Curl the toes under with the in-breath.

❷ Exhale and lift the hips up and back as you straighten the legs. Breathe in the pose for a short time. Bend the knees and come down. Rest in Child Pose, and repeat.

Child Pose and Downward Facing Dog are a sequence—try three cycles. Hold the first Downward Facing Dog for a short time, rest in Child Pose, and gradually increase the time held in the second and third sequence.

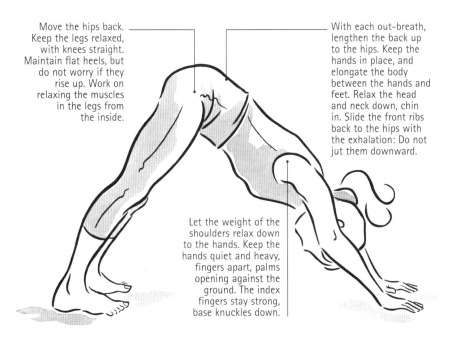

Move the hips back. Keep the legs relaxed, with knees straight. Maintain flat heels, but do not worry if they rise up. Work on relaxing the muscles in the legs from the inside.

With each out-breath, lengthen the back up to the hips. Keep the hands in place, and elongate the body between the hands and feet. Relax the head and neck down, chin in. Slide the front ribs back to the hips with the exhalation: Do not jut them downward.

Let the weight of the shoulders relax down to the hands. Keep the hands quiet and heavy, fingers apart, palms opening against the ground. The index fingers stay strong, base knuckles down.

pranayama (BREATHING)

Prana is Sanskrit for both "breath" and "universal life force," while *ayama* means "control." Sitting and breathing for five minutes a day will help improve your concentration and make you feel more relaxed. If five minutes seems an unbearable amount of time, try for one minute. Indeed, as a beginner, you shouldn't work for more than five minutes at first.

When you feel comfortable in your chosen sitting position, relax your shoulders and bend your arms at the elbow. Rest your hands on your thighs, palms up. Keep your back straight, the back of your neck long, and your head upright, chin in. Relax your face, keeping your expression calm and eyes closed.

sitting positions

To breathe easily, you need to be comfortable and stable. Sit cross-legged or try one of these positions: On a chair with back straight and thighs horizontal (place a cushion beneath them on a low chair or books beneath your feet on a high chair); or on the ground with back against a wall, a small cushion between the base of your spine, and the wall and legs crossed or straight and apart (place a cushion under each knee).

ujjayi (SIMPLE BREATHING)

Visualize the breath traveling down the inside of the spine. Allow the breath to settle into its own rhythm. Exhale, starting at the back of your throat, and moving down your body. Inhale, starting at the base of your belly and moving back up your body. Keep shoulders still.

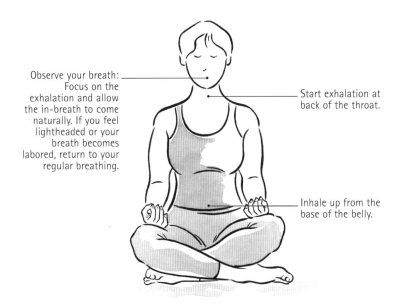

Observe your breath: Focus on the exhalation and allow the in-breath to come naturally. If you feel lightheaded or your breath becomes labored, return to your regular breathing.

Start exhalation at back of the throat.

Inhale up from the base of the belly.

relaxation

After each yoga session, lie down for 5 or 10 minutes. Relaxation after practicing poses and pranayama smooths out any strain, protecting against muscle stiffness. Lie on a blanket or a non-slip mat. Place a blanket over you, or wear a warm-up suit and socks, to keep warm. If you find lying on the ground uncomfortable or you have respiratory problems, place a pillow under your head. If your back is tense, elevate your lower legs on a chair for the exercise.

recuperation pose I

❶ Lie on the ground with knees bent and feet flat on the floor. Keep the back of the pelvis flat. Place your arms on either side of you, palms facing up. Close your eyes. Let your breath settle into its own rhythm. Gradually focus more on the out-breath: Exhale down the body and let the in-breath return up the body.

❷ Relax the shoulders; keep the hips wide and heavy. Exhale, feeling the ground beneath you and your body against it.

savasana (CORPSE POSE)

Start in Recuperation Pose *(see opposite)*, then lengthen your legs out along the ground.

❶ Breathe out into the back of the waist to relax the lower back; feel the heaviness of the back of the legs.

❷ Relax the face and jaw. Keep the shoulders relaxed and the hips wide and heavy.

❸ Exhale a little deeper, and let the in-breath come easily. Feel where your body touches the ground; relax against it.

❹ After three cycles of conscious breath, open the eyes, roll to one side, stretch, and get up slowly.

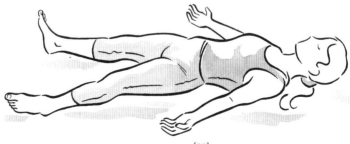

the story of yoga

Yoga might have had roots in other countries. However, if we take the religious history of India, we can see how yoga became part of the development of a culture. Indian philosophy has always been concerned with questions on the meaning of the existence of human beings. Questions like: Why are we here? and Where are we going? are as relevant today as they were then.

The way in which these questions were considered was through introspection. Yoga encouraged introspection through concentration and meditation. Through using techniques of breath control, meditation was transcended into other states. Shamanism, the earliest of magic religious beliefs, also used states of altered consciousness to enter other realms of reality populated by spirits. There is evidence of both shamanistic beliefs and yogic practices in the earliest known civilization which had established itself by c.2250 BC. This was the Harappan Civilization.

In the North West of the Indian subcontinent, in what is now Pakistan, two main cities, Harappa and Mohenjo-daro were built in the valley of the Indus River. Through controlling the flooding of the waters of the Indus, a sustainable agriculture was provided for a large community which covered 1000 miles from the Arabian Sea to the foothills of the Himalayas. The Harappan Civilization was contemporary with that of Mesopotamia and trade, via the Persian Gulf, existed between the two.

Goods were shipped from the port of Lothal, wrapped in linen with terracotta seals on which were depicted animals and gods. One of the most famous seals has the figure of a god seated in a yoga position. He wears a headdress of horns and is surrounded by four animals, a rhinoceros, a tiger, a water buffalo and an elephant. He is thought to be an early representation of the Hindu god, Shiva, who was also known as Lord of the Beasts (Pashu-pati) and Lord of yoga.

The Harappan religion contained priests, gods and animal sacrifice. They revered cows, bulls and snakes and a goddess and male fertility god were worshipped. Harappa and Mohenjo-daro were built from burnt bricks, an advance on the porous sundried ones, and had wide streets, drainage systems and houses with bathrooms which suggests ritual ablutions similar to modern Hinduism.

In c.1750BC the Indo-European tribes of Aryans began to invade from the north but the city cultures were already in decline. There was military violence for the Aryans were warriors but the decline could also have been from natural changes to the flooding of the Indus or through de-forestation from the firing of the brick kilns.

month2

In this, your second month of yoga practice, the main posture for contemplation is Tree Pose, a balance on one leg, and apt for the season of spring, signifying, as it does, a wonderful upward growth that refreshes body and mind. The subject for the month is gravity, and Tree Pose enhances the sense of balance and rootedness established in month 1 to help counter the negative effects of gravity on the body. Many of the other asanas offered in this sequence also encourage flexibility and grounding principles, including supine poses and sitting poses. Breathing exercises continue to work on Ujjayi, or simple breathing.

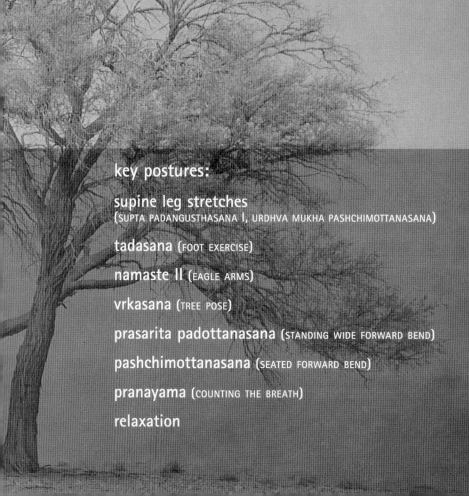

key postures:

supine leg stretches
(SUPTA PADANGUSTHASANA I, URDHVA MUKHA PASHCHIMOTTANASANA)

tadasana (FOOT EXERCISE)

namaste II (EAGLE ARMS)

vrkasana (TREE POSE)

prasarita padottanasana (STANDING WIDE FORWARD BEND)

pashchimottanasana (SEATED FORWARD BEND)

pranayama (COUNTING THE BREATH)

relaxation

gravity and confidence

A tree stays upright by its network of roots that spreads out and pulls downward. Similarly, the body must develop a feeling of being pulled down into the ground. The tree grows upward toward the sky, and the body, too, relies on a two-way movement at the back of the waist to maintain balance, lengthening the spine upward with the breath as weight drops down toward the feet.

The force of gravity pulls toward the center of the earth, but it also has a rebounding energy, an anti-force, that springs back up. As your foot presses into the ground, an energy returns through the body from this contact, releasing upward.

Most people when balancing on two legs feel confident that they won't fall. Even so, trips and slips happen, usually at absent-minded moments. Standing on one leg requires concentration and steadiness of mind, and learning to steady the mind with yoga boosts confidence: The confidence not to fall and general confidence, too, because if the mind is focused, it is easier to see what is around you.

Lying down at the start of a yoga session helps to re-focus a busy mind and relaxes the hips and shoulders. First settle the breath with the exercise opposite, then warm the body with the supine leg stretches on pages 34-35.

Recuperation Pose II

❶ Lie on the floor as illustrated, eyes open. Let your breathing settle into its own rhythm.

❷ After letting an in-breath come, exhale deeply down the body.

❸ Breathe out to the back of the waist, lengthening down to the tailbone and up to the crown of the head. Repeat several times.

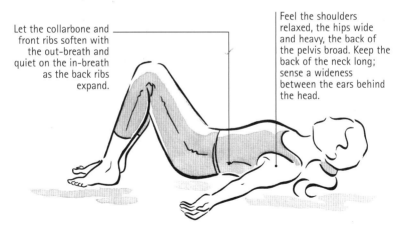

Let the collarbone and front ribs soften with the out-breath and quiet on the in-breath as the back ribs expand.

Feel the shoulders relaxed, the hips wide and heavy, the back of the pelvis broad. Keep the back of the neck long; sense a wideness between the ears behind the head.

supine leg stretches

To encourage the hamstrings to release, and to ease backpain, these poses can be done against a wall. Do not leave your legs up for too long: They may go numb.

supta padangusthasana I
(SINGLE LEG STRETCH)

❶ From Recuperation Pose II (page 33) lie on your back, knees bent, and bring the right knee to your chest. Hold beneath the knee. Straighten the left leg along the floor.

❷ Direct the exhalation into the fold of the right leg, and draw the knee in. Relax on the in-breath. Repeat.

❸ Exhale and extend the right leg until straight. Loop a belt around the foot and hold with the right hand in the loop.

❹ Toward the end of the out-breath, draw the right leg to you. Relax on the in-breath. After some breath cycles, repeat from step 1 on the other leg.

urdhva mukha pashchimottanasana

(SUPINE DOUBLE LEG STRETCH)

Fold both knees in toward your chest and hold above or
below the knees. Breathe out into the folds of the hips,
drawing the knees in. On an exhalation, extend your legs
upward. If you're flexible, hold your feet with your hands;
if not, loop a belt over the feet. Keep your legs straight
and the back of the pelvis and tailbone down.

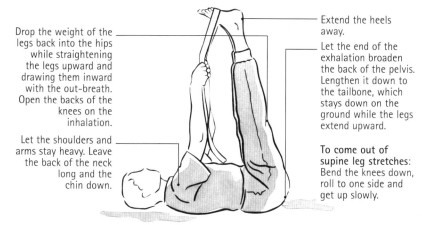

Drop the weight of the
legs back into the hips
while straightening
the legs upward and
drawing them inward
with the out-breath.
Open the backs of the
knees on the
inhalation.

Let the shoulders and
arms stay heavy. Leave
the back of the neck
long and the
chin down.

Extend the heels
away.

Let the end of the
exhalation broaden
the back of the pelvis.
Lengthen it down to
the tailbone, which
stays down on the
ground while the legs
extend upward.

**To come out of
supine leg stretches:**
Bend the knees down,
roll to one side and
get up slowly.

tadasana (FOOT EXERCISE)

The foot absorbs compression when you walk, run, or jump through its padded sole and arches. The toes can be almost as mobile as fingers, and were when we were babies. Use this exercise to mobilize the toes, raise the arches, and bring a spring to your step!

❶ Stand in Tadasana *(see pages 14-15)* and relax the toes.

❷ Leaving the balls of the feet down, raise all the toes. Relax and repeat.

❸ Leave the big toe and little toe of each foot down on the ground, and raise the three toes in between.
If the message from the brain isn't getting through (it's a long way to the feet and not a message often sent), bend the knees and hold down the big and little toes while raising the three toes in between.

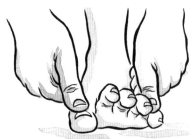

namaste II (EAGLE ARMS)

Prepare for this exercise by standing and swinging your arms gently. Repeat the whole exercise on both sides.

❶ Exhale and place the right elbow in the crook of the left elbow, the backs of the arms together.

❷ Wrap the hands around each other so that the palms are facing one another.

❸ Feel a stretch across the back of the shoulders. As you exhale, take the arms up, feeling the stretch increase. Do not strain or force the shoulders. Make room in the shoulders from the inside with the breath.

❹ Relax the arms down, shake the wrists gently to get rid of tension.

vrkasana (TREE POSE)

This asana is like a tree that keeps its roots in the earth while the branches grow upward. When balancing, feel the vertical action of gravity drawing you straighter over your supporting leg. If the balance is difficult, place your hand on the back of a chair. Fold the knee in nearest the chair as this improves straightness and balance over the supporting leg.

❶ Stand in Tadasana *(see pages 14-15)* and feel the weight evenly in both feet before taking the weight onto the left leg.

❷ Exhale and bend the right knee up, placing the foot on the opposite inner leg. To get it higher, hold the ankle, and move the foot up. If the foot slips down, support it by holding it with a belt around the ankle.

❸ Exhale and take the arms into Namaste (prayer position). Let the in-breath come easily. If you feel ready, raise the arms above the head. Breathe, developing the pose, then repeat all the steps on the right leg.

In Tree Pose, everything below the waist sinks down, while the upper body lengthens up with the exhalation.

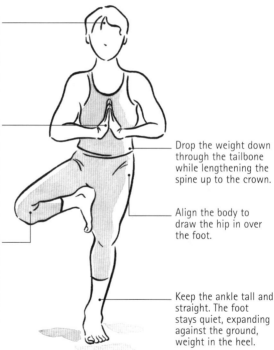

Focus concentration in the eyes, keeping them level and looking to the middle distance. Lengthen the back of the neck, bringing the chin in.

Place the hands in Namaste (prayer position), lower arms down, palms together, and hands a little way from the body. If you are stable, take the arms above the head, apart or in Namaste.

Rotate the hip outward so that the sole of the foot is flat against the standing leg. The bent knee is heavy, pressing the heel in, and the inner thigh is strong in return against the foot.

Drop the weight down through the tailbone while lengthening the spine up to the crown.

Align the body to draw the hip in over the foot.

Keep the ankle tall and straight. The foot stays quiet, expanding against the ground, weight in the heel.

prasarita padottanasana

(STANDING WIDE FORWARD BEND)

This asana is based in the strong triangle of the legs and
feet. From this base, the spine releases away from the hips
and lengthens forward. The weight of the hips and legs
drops down to the feet. Hold the pose for as long as is
comfortable. Use a non-slip mat; this allows you to drop
your weight without the outside feet being over-strong. As
with other forward bends, you can use a chair to start with.

❶ Stand in Tadasana *(see pages 14-15)*, then take the feet
apart. To begin with, don't take the legs too wide. Keep
the toes pointing inward to stop the feet from slipping.

❷ Exhale and bend forward from the hips. As the in-
breath comes, do nothing. When the stomach contracts
toward the end of the next out-breath, let the lower back
lengthen and the spine extend forward and down.

❸ As the hands come down, take them back to continue
lengthening the spine.

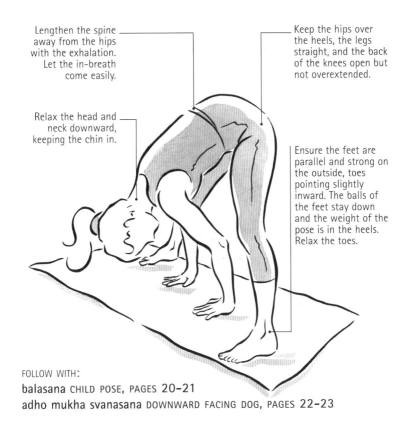

Lengthen the spine away from the hips with the exhalation. Let the in-breath come easily.

Keep the hips over the heels, the legs straight, and the back of the knees open but not overextended.

Relax the head and neck downward, keeping the chin in.

Ensure the feet are parallel and strong on the outside, toes pointing slightly inward. The balls of the feet stay down and the weight of the pose is in the heels. Relax the toes.

FOLLOW WITH:
balasana CHILD POSE, PAGES 20–21
adho mukha svanasana DOWNWARD FACING DOG, PAGES 22–23

pashchimottanasana

(SEATED FORWARD BEND)

The sitting bones, the boney bits in the buttocks, are the roots of this pose. These remain heavy while the spine lengthens up and forward with the exhalation. Because it is symmetrical, this asana makes a good end to this month's yoga routine. It is also a soothing pose, the spine releasing as the pelvis rotates forward at the hips.

The ability to bend forward relies on looseness in the hamstrings. If tight, they stop the pelvis from rotating and leave the spine hunched. If you have disk problems or tight hamstrings you can do the pose going forward to the seat of a chair placed over the legs. Rest your head and arms on the seat, breathing into the back to lengthen it, and leaving the base of the pose heavy.

❶ First settle yourself. Place the hands on the ground behind, fingers toward the feet, and relax. Sit upright, feeling the sitting bones against the ground beneath you.

❷ Exhale, lengthening forward from the hips. Develop with the breath as long as is comfortable.

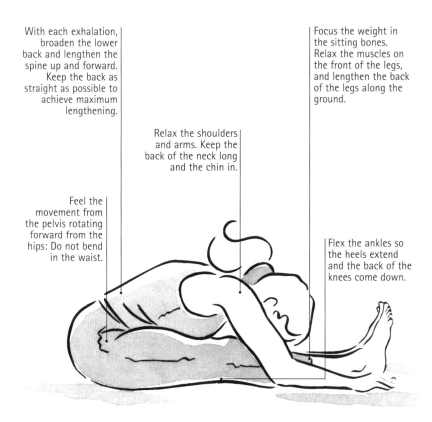

With each exhalation, broaden the lower back and lengthen the spine up and forward. Keep the back as straight as possible to achieve maximum lengthening.

Focus the weight in the sitting bones. Relax the muscles on the front of the legs, and lengthen the back of the legs along the ground.

Relax the shoulders and arms. Keep the back of the neck long and the chin in.

Feel the movement from the pelvis rotating forward from the hips: Do not bend in the waist.

Flex the ankles so the heels extend and the back of the knees come down.

pranayama (COUNTING THE BREATH)

Practice Pranayama for 5 minutes. According to how you
sat in month 1 *(see page 25)*, progress gradually to sitting
cross-legged without the support of the wall.

❶ Place the palms on the ground behind you, fingers
facing feet, and relax the legs. Stretch up and bend
forward. Exhale toward the sitting bones, lengthening the
lower back, then return upright.

❷ Close the eyes and rest the hands on the knees or thighs,
palms up. Relax the face, straighten the spine and drop the
upper-body weight to the sitting bones. Allow the breath to
quieten and practice Ujjayi breathing *(see page 25)*.

❸ Select a number like 5, or 6 and, in your mind, count
from that number down through the out-breath and up
through the in-breath. Don't alter anything, just observe
and return to Ujjayi breathing. Repeat several cycles. On
another day, using your selected number, make the
exhalation and the inhalation even. Repeat for several
cycles and return to Ujjayi breathing.

relaxation

Start by lying in Recuperation Pose I *(see page 26)* and breathe easily until you feel your body relax against the ground. Then lengthen your legs out into Savasana *(see page 29)*. If, as the legs straighten, the lower back suddenly pops up, breathe out into the back of the waist and let it relax.

❶ Follow the breath as it goes down the path of the inside of the spine. Be aware of the start of the out-breath, at the back of the throat.

❷ Relax the face and jaw, especially where the jaw hinges beneath the ears.

❸ Breathe out a little deeper and observe how the in-breath comes naturally. Feel the ground beneath you and be aware of your body against the ground.

❹ After five conscious cycles of breathing, open the eyes, roll to one side, stretch, and slowly get up.

the story of yoga

By the time the nomadic Aryans came from beyond the Hindu Kush, the peaceful urban population of the Indus Valley was not able to repel them. The invaders were warriors with horse-drawn chariots and bronze weapons. They were also cattle people, in contrast to the pastoral agricultural society of the Harappans, and were greedy for grazing land.

Aryan is a linguistic term for Indo-European people from tribes originating in the southern steppes of Russia. They were strong and confident, fearing only their enemy's magic spells. They did not have a sophisticated culture like the urban valley dwellers, but held deep religious beliefs. A pantheon of gods fought with the solar light of truth against the forces of darkness. Their gods represented the forces of nature, and stories about them were sung and recited as poetry until they were collected in a series of incantations and hymns, ancient rules and lore, known as the Vedas, "Books of Knowledge." There are four Vedas: The Rigveda composed before 1200 B.C.E.; the Samaveda; the Yajurveda; and the later Atharvaveda.

Traditional belief has it that the hymns were composed by seers (rishis) in a state of contemplation during the ritual of sacrifice. The yoga in the Vedas is characterized by concentration, watchfulness, austerities, and regulation of the breath within the incantation, like a sound mantra. The sacred syllables, from which gods and mortals were born, included "aum," whose vibration was thought to have created the universe.

Sacrifice was the main ceremony for the Vedic-Aryans, who did not have buildings for worship or idols. Their priests (Brahmins) were concerned, to begin with, solely in these rites. It was through sacrifice that the gods were invoked and appeased. The sacrificial area was a sphere of purity in what the Brahmin priests considered to be an impure world. Later, there was an aversion to killing within this area, and eventually the killing became symbolic.

The Vedic-Aryans spoke Sanskrit, and in the hymns there is evidence of their own pre-history of shamanistic beliefs. When they first arrived in the Indus Valley, these nomadic tribes worshiped Varuna, a deity who ruled the universe and was the moral ruler of cosmic order (Rita). Varuna was a frightening and wrathful god who was superseded by Indra as king of the gods.

Indra, god of rain and thunder, had heroic qualities, and was a warrior of action. In his victory over Vritra, a symbol of chaos, the invaders saw a metaphor of their struggle against the inhabitants of the Indus Valley. Such stories changed as the invaders settled and assimilated local beliefs.

month3

In the third and last month of spring, time of new beginnings, your body will be feeling stronger and more renewed, being more accustomed to yoga practice. Capitalize on this sensation with the main pose for study, the Warrior, a symbol of power and stamina in Indian mythology. The thought of the month concerns motion—the exchange of weight through the body, as in walking or running. At the end of the yoga sequence, use the refreshing breathing exercises to develop the simple Ujjayi breath further.

key postures:

warming up (SUPTA VRAJRASANA)

vajrasana (THUNDERBOLT POSE)

parivrtta vajrasana (TWISTING THUNDERBOLT)

eka pada rajakapotasana I (ONE LEGGED PIGEON POSE Î)

virabhadrasana (WARRIOR POSE)

parivrtta janu shirshasana I (TWISTING HEAD-TO-KNEE)

pranayama (SIGHING BREATH)

relaxation

losing and finding

Walking, learned at an early age, takes many years to perfect. A toddler's method is to roll the body from side to side, keeping the base wide to prevent falls as the weight moves from leg to leg.

The toddler is right to be careful, because walking is a constant process of falling and saving oneself. The foot pressed against the ground pushes the body up and forward, toppling it, before it is caught by the next step.

Often in walking, the chin gets to the destination first, the legs drag behind, and walking is tiring. There is a saying, "Don't put the cart before the horse." If the horse pushed the cart, it would take a great deal of effort, and the cart would bump into every stone in the road. In walking, the legs resemble the horse—the motive force—that goes first, while the body is the cart that follows after.

In a perfect walking motion, the head, with eyes to navigate, and the body are upright, staying over the center of gravity of whichever foot is on the ground. The heel goes down first so that the whole length of the foot can be used and adapt to the ground. As the foot pushes against the ground, energy rebounds, and motion takes the body forward. Walking becomes effortless, the last step is lost and the next found.

warming up

Start with the two supine leg stretches on pages 34–35.
Try practicing the double leg stretch first and the single
stretches after. Follow these with Lying Down Diamond
(see below), a very gentle pose that warms and relaxes the
body for the sequence of poses to come.

supta vrajrasana

(LYING DOWN DIAMOND)

❶ Lying on your back, bend the knees onto the chest,
leaving the arms on the ground. Cross the ankles.

❷ Rock gently from side to side, making sure the
shoulders stay on the floor.

❸ Cross the ankles the opposite way and rock gently
again, massaging the back of the pelvis.

vajrasana (THUNDERBOLT POSE)

Thunderbolt is a powerful name for a pose and refers to the weapon of Indra, king of the gods in Hindu mythology. A strong, stable kneeling position, it is also known as Diamond, and can be seen in Egyptian wall paintings. Thunderbolt is a good pose in which to practice breathing and meditation: Because the pelvis is straight, the spine is able to find its line of balance. If uncomfortable, place a cushion under the thighs and a rolled blanket under the tops of the feet. Follow the steps below, then move on to the Thunderbolt Twist, opposite.

❶ Kneel with the heels beneath the sitting bones, pelvis straight. Feel the spine align up from the pelvis.

❷ Feet exercise: Turn the toes under and sit back on heels, stretch the feet and toes. If painful, don't hold for long, but repeat a couple of times. Also try turning the toes on each foot under separately. Bring one knee up and sit back on the other foot. This benefits the feet, enlivening them and increasing flexibility.

parivrtta vajrasana

(THUNDERBOLT TWIST)

Still kneeling in Vajrasana *(see step 1 opposite)*, take it into Parivrtta Vajrasana, a simple twist.

❶ Exhale and turn to one side, the arms going with the movement. Remain in this position for several cycles of breath, letting yourself become more comfortable.

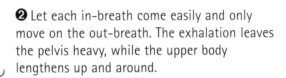

❷ Let each in-breath come easily and only move on the out-breath. The exhalation leaves the pelvis heavy, while the upper body lengthens up and around.

❸ Feel the spiralling of the upper back in the twist, and let the shoulder blades move toward each other. As the pelvis is kept straight by its weight and the legs beneath, it is not as easy to feel the twist coming from the base of the spine. Repeat all the steps, turning the other way.

[53]

eka pada rajakapotasana I

(ONE LEGGED PIGEON POSE I)

It is good to include this pose in your practice to warm the hips and increase their flexibility. It also helps ease lower-back pain. The first stage of a more advanced pose, it is like a static version of leaping hurdles. Directing the out-breath to any tightness or tension is a useful lesson that began with the single supine leg stretches *(see pages 34–35)*. Here, feel how the out-breath goes deeper.

❶ Kneeling on hands and knees, take the right knee forward. The thigh stays in line with the right side of the body, and the knee points toward the right armpit.

❷ Bring the right lower leg obliquely across under the body so the outside of the foot is on the floor by the left hip.

❸ Lengthen the left leg behind, arms in front to stop the body sinking down quickly. Exhale into the stretch at the top back of the right thigh to help the muscles release. If the knee strains, do not sink down. Repeat on the other leg, then change sides a few times.

Keep the left side of the upper body straight and in line with the right thigh.

Rest the arms and forehead on the ground, shoulders relaxed.

Let the back of the pelvis stay wide and drop the weight down beneath the right hip. Exhale into the furthest point of the turning hip. Let the in-breath come easily.

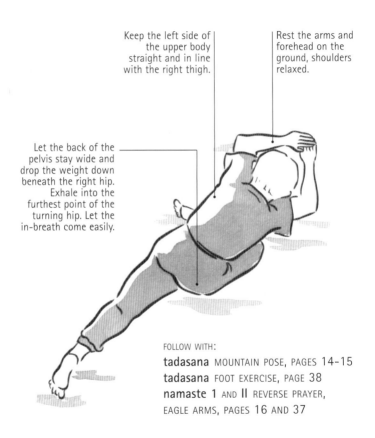

FOLLOW WITH:

tadasana MOUNTAIN POSE, PAGES 14–15
tadasana FOOT EXERCISE, PAGE 38
namaste 1 AND II REVERSE PRAYER,
EAGLE ARMS, PAGES 16 AND 37

virabhadrasana (WARRIOR POSE)

Warrior Pose exchanges body weight from back to front foot. Test this by stepping forward with one foot and bending the knee; take the weight forward and back. The front leg bends and straightens as it receives the weight; the back heel moves up and down, like walking. Keep the body straight above the foot with the weight.

1 From Tadasana *(see pages 14–15)*, take the weight onto the right leg. With the left leg, step forward one pace, and bend the knee. Keep the weight over the back heel.

2 Exhale, and take the arms up. Keep the shoulders down and weight over the back heel, hip and body straight above.

3 Exhale; transfer weight to the front foot. Straighten the knee and drop the weight into the front heel, body above.

4 Exhale and hinge at the hip, body moving forward, arms and back leg aligned, heel extended. Repeat on the right leg.

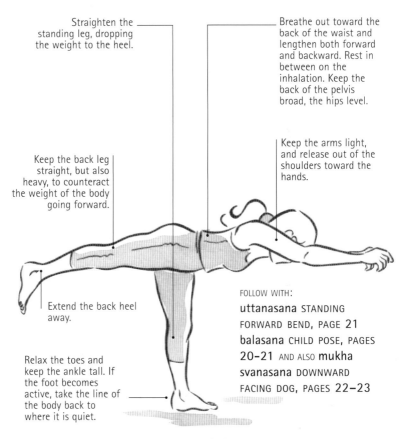

Straighten the standing leg, dropping the weight to the heel.

Breathe out toward the back of the waist and lengthen both forward and backward. Rest in between on the inhalation. Keep the back of the pelvis broad, the hips level.

Keep the arms light, and release out of the shoulders toward the hands.

Keep the back leg straight, but also heavy, to counteract the weight of the body going forward.

Extend the back heel away.

Relax the toes and keep the ankle tall. If the foot becomes active, take the line of the body back to where it is quiet.

FOLLOW WITH:

uttanasana STANDING FORWARD BEND, PAGE 21 **balasana** CHILD POSE, PAGES 20–21 AND ALSO **mukha svanasana** DOWNWARD FACING DOG, PAGES 22–23

parivrtta janu shirshasana I

(TWISTING HEAD-TO-KNEE)

This is the first stage of this pose, an open twist in which the sitting bones at the base of the pelvis are as important to grounding the body as the feet are in standing poses.

❶ Sit on the ground and lengthen the left leg. Bend the right knee at an angle, sole of the foot facing the left leg.

❷ To settle yourself, place your hands on the ground behind, fingers facing the feet, and let the legs relax. Extend up and feel the weight in the sitting bones.

❸ Exhale and turn to the right. Take time, so that each out-breath helps the turn, the ribs sliding gently around. Take the right arm around the back of the waist, resting the left arm on the right thigh. If you feel unstable, place your right hand on the ground behind.

❹ Develop the pose, letting the spine turn, then repeat the twist on the other side.

Twists work from the base of the spine upward. The sitting bones stay heavy, anchored to the ground.

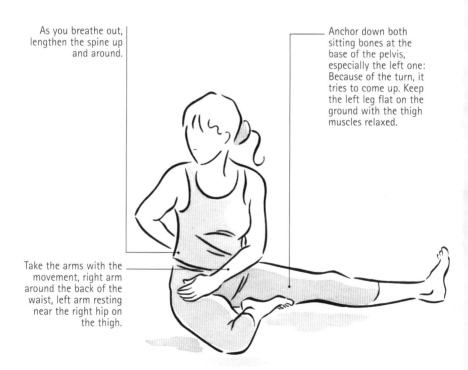

As you breathe out, lengthen the spine up and around.

Anchor down both sitting bones at the base of the pelvis, especially the left one: Because of the turn, it tries to come up. Keep the left leg flat on the ground with the thigh muscles relaxed.

Take the arms with the movement, right arm around the back of the waist, left arm resting near the right hip on the thigh.

pranayama

(SIGHING BREATH)

The first two months of spring focused on Ujjayi breathing *(see page 25)* to observe how you, yourself, breathe. This month introduces a longer out-breath. Continue moving toward sitting cross-legged without support, changing the cross of your legs when uncomfortable.

❶ Settle with hands behind you and legs relaxed. Exhale, lengthening forward from the lower back. Return upright. Close your eyes and rest the hands on the knees, palms up. Let your breathing settle, then focus on the out-breath, allowing the in-breath to come naturally.

❷ After the in-breath, sigh, exhaling strongly to the bottom of the breath. At the end of the out-breath, the abdomen contracts toward the backbone. Relax the abdomen and let the in-breath come easily, then sigh again. Repeat three times, then return to Ujjayi breathing. When relaxed, repeat the sigh three times, letting the in-breath come between. Return to Ujjayi breathing, then lie down.

relaxation

Lie in Recuperation Pose I *(see page 26)* with eyes closed. Breathe easily until your body relaxes against the ground, then lengthen the legs into Savasana *(see page 27)*. Exhale toward the back of the waist to relax and lengthen it. Keep the shoulders relaxed, and hips wide.

❶ Feel the weight of the body and the ground where it touches it. As you exhale, give the weight of the body to the solid, supportive ground.

❷ Let each out-breath relax the back of the body against the ground, letting the floor support you more and more.

❸ Relax the face, jaw, and forehead. As the out-breath goes down the back of the throat, feel it drop down the inside of the spine, behind the front ribs and the stomach. At the bottom, note the in-breath starting to come back up the body, widening the ribs on the sides and back.

❹ After five conscious breath cycles, open the eyes, roll to one side, and get up slowly.

the story of yoga

Between the 7th and 5th centuries B.C.E., the early texts of the Upanishads were composed. They are the last texts of the Vedas and are known as the Vedanta or Conclusion of the Vedas. The tone of these treatises and poems is philosophical and mystical, and there is no longer an interest in ritual sacrifice. While the Vedas were hymns to the outer world of creation, to nature and its forces, the Upanishads provide a transformation of thought, in which the Divine or transcending principle is searched for from within. The self-training for this is yoga.

The Upanishads, like the Vedas, were not written down to begin with, but memorized and handed down from teacher to pupil. The Sanskrit term upanishad refers to sitting for instruction at the feet of a master, and the Sanskrit word guru means a spiritual teacher. This method of transferring knowledge by teaching yoga on a one-to-one basis has been employed up to the present day. However, increased communication and translation of the texts are now changing this approach.

The teaching of the Upanishads was concerned with the desire for release (moksha) from the round of births and deaths through reincarnation that had been accepted as a concept by the time of the Upanishads' conception. This release, the writings taught, was to be gained through meditation, yoga, and asceticism, which would unite the soul (atman) within with the absolute spirit (brahman) without.

The concept of karma, by which every action, good or bad, has a cause and therefore a reaction that is impossible to escape, was also accepted. Because of reincarnation, it is believed, actions in our present lives determine our fate in lives that follow through the karmic memory in our higher consciousness. Desire is the cause of karma and, because of the desire to live in the ordinary world, the cycle of samsara, the endless chain of rebirth, cannot be escaped. Actions without desires for reward or attainment free the soul from the effects of karma.

The thoughts contained in the Upanishads, counteracting the ritualism of the Vedas, were enormously influential. By 500 B.C.E., religion and society were changing. Cities had begun to grow again, and a strong merchant class was upsetting the old orders of priest, warrior, trader, and serf. The Vedic-Aryans had taken over northern India, and the center of their culture was in the north-eastern delta of the Ganges.

An aggressive empire of the Maghada dynasty led a number of disaffected groups to follow their own paths of beliefs away from the increasingly rigid interpretation of the Brahmin priests. Breakaway sects of ascetics, mystics, and renunciants began to follow new teachers, such as Siddartha Gautoma (c.563–483 B.C.E.), the Buddha, and Vardhamana (c.599–527 B.C.E.), who became the Mahavira and founded Jainism.

section I index

summer

growth

With the blossom of summer comes your unfurling growth. The next three months of yoga routines develop standing, sitting, and kneeling postures. Intersperse these sequences with the simpler routines of the first three months, and notice how much you have progressed. Always start with the supine warming-up stretches and you will find you are ready for the heat and high energy of summer.

month 4
month 5
month 6

month4

The first month of asanas for summer introduces the Triangle Poses, which tap your hidden reserves of energy and vitality, and offer a new sense of direction. The focus for thought is standing and turning. There are also more twists and Bridge Pose, a half backarch and the first of the highly energizing and rejuvenating backbends. Breathing focuses on the interval pause, a crystal-clear moment of suspension that offers an opening that is quite special.

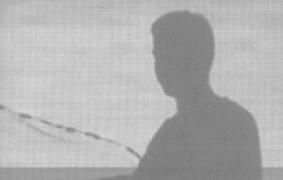

key postures:

warming up (JATARA PARIVARTANASANA I)

trikonasana (TRIANGLE POSE)

parsva konasana (SIDE ANGLE POSE)

setu bandha sarvangasana (BRIDGE POSE-HALF BACKARCH)

jatara parivartanasana II (SUPINE TWIST II)

janu shirshasana (SEATED HEAD-TO-KNEE)

upavistha konasana (OPEN ANGLE)

pranayama (VILOMA-INTERVAL BREATHING ON THE OUT-BREATH)

relaxation

spirals and turning

The practice of yoga is like a spiral. It is a continual development that passes from yesterday's discoveries to today's. The yoga you learns stays with you, and, once learned, the knowledge increases. This doesn't mean that basic principles are not looked at again; rather, that in re-examination, the basics produce new meanings.

The pace of a spiral is regulated by the way it turns around the center, not aiming directly at it, but curving around. Similarly, in yoga, the approach to a pose is circular, investigatory. A pose is not finalized, but continues to reveal. If this were not true, there would be no need to practice an asana again. It is wise to be circular in approaching poses, not homing in directly on a perceived center that may not be there, but moving around, looking from all sides, going away, and coming back.

In standing and turning poses, the upper back and shoulders become more flexible. The pelvis and legs provide the base for the turn to release from. To balance the upper and lower spine, the backbone starts its turn from the base of the spine, and works upward, smoothing the process and helping to prevent uneven pressure. The exhalation protects and elongates the spine, making the spiralling motion more apparent. Turning to look behind easily is also turning to look all around.

warming up

Lie in Recuperation Pose II *(see page 33)*. Then do the supine leg stretches on pages 34–35 and Supine Twist I *(see below)*.

jatara parivartanasana I
(SUPINE TWIST I)

❶ Start in Recuperation Pose II *(see page 33)*. Leaving the shoulders flat, exhale and roll the knees and pelvis to one side. On another exhalation bring them back to the center.

❷ Exhale and roll the knees and pelvis to the other side. Repeat a few times, moving the legs on the out-breath.

❸ As the knees roll one way, let the head and neck roll the other. Repeat a couple of times to both sides, always moving on the out-breath.

FOLLOW WITH: tadasana MOUNTAIN POSE, PAGE 15, tadasana FEET EXERCISES PAGE 38 AND namaste REVERSED PRAYER, PAGE 18

namaste III

(BHUJA GOMUKHASANA—COW ARMS)

This is an excellent opener for the shoulders and arms.
One side is usually easier to practice on than the other.

1 Take the right arm above the head, relax the shoulder
down, bend the arm at the elbow and drop it behind the
neck, palm inward.

2 Exhale and take the left arm behind the back, palm
facing outward.

3 Move the hands towards each other until
the fingers can clasp each other. If the hands
don't touch, hold a belt in the upper
hand and bring the other arm round to
catch it. Gradually work the hands
toward each other.

4 Drop the arms down, shake the
wrists gently, and repeat the stretch
on the other side.

trikonasana (TRIANGLE POSE)

The next asana in this month's sequence boosts flexibility in the hips and shoulders and also benefits the eyes. The pose starts from Tadasana *(see pages 14–15)* and has two stages, illustrated on pages 72–73. During your practice, always keep your weight in the back leg.

❶ From Tadasana *(see pages 14–15)*, step forward, keeping the weight over the back heel.

❷ TRIANGLE STAGE 1 Exhale and turn toward the back foot. Extend the arm out behind and look along the arm toward the hand *(see illustration, page 72)*. Stay here, breathing for a few cycles, grounding the back heel and feeling the upper body lengthen upward and around in the turn.

❸ TRIANGLE STAGE 2 Exhale, keep the weight in the back heel, and lengthen the spine sideways away from the back hip, letting the back arm come up. Relax the front arm downward and look up toward the top hand *(see illustration, page 73)*.

❹ Develop for a few cycles of breath then return upright.

trikonasana

(TRIANGLE POSE, STAGE 1)

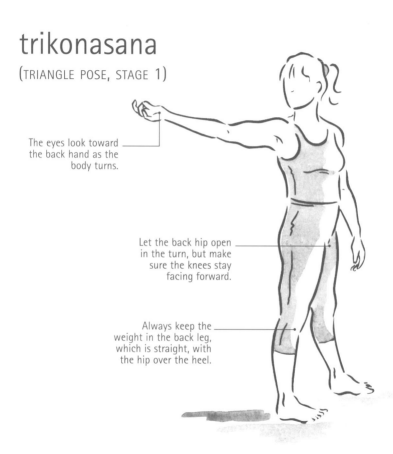

The eyes look toward the back hand as the body turns.

Let the back hip open in the turn, but make sure the knees stay facing forward.

Always keep the weight in the back leg, which is straight, with the hip over the heel.

(TRIANGLE POSE, STAGE 2)

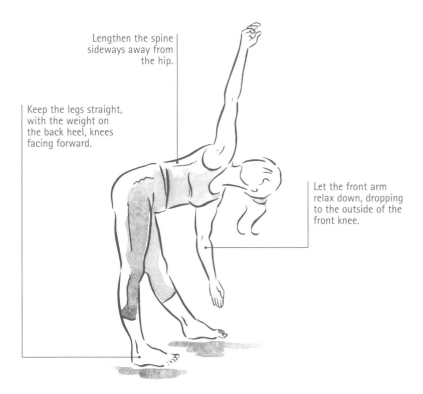

Lengthen the spine sideways away from the hip.

Keep the legs straight, with the weight on the back heel, knees facing forward.

Let the front arm relax down, dropping to the outside of the front knee.

parsva konasana (SIDE ANGLE POSE)

The movements of this pose are the same as Trikonasana but the front leg is bent at the knee. It is easier to go further forward, but harder to keep the knees, especially the front knee, facing forward. Only go as far forward as the weight in the back heel against the ground allows and so that breathing can be maintained with ease.

❶ From Tadasana *(Mountain Pose, see page 15)*, take the weight on to the right leg and step forward with the left, leaving the knee bent.

❷ Exhale and turn to the right, taking the right arm out behind and looking toward it. Breathe a few cycles of breath while establishing the weight in the back heel and until you feel comfortable in the turn.

❸ Exhale and lengthen sideways and forward. The right arm follows the movement upward while the left drops to the outside of the knee. Look up toward the arm on an exhalation, and with the back heel anchoring you firmly, come upright. Repeat on the other side.

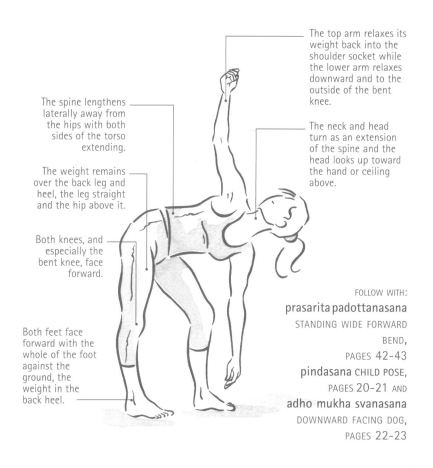

The top arm relaxes its weight back into the shoulder socket while the lower arm relaxes downward and to the outside of the bent knee.

The spine lengthens laterally away from the hips with both sides of the torso extending.

The neck and head turn as an extension of the spine and the head looks up toward the hand or ceiling above.

The weight remains over the back leg and heel, the leg straight and the hip above it.

Both knees, and especially the bent knee, face forward.

Both feet face forward with the whole of the foot against the ground, the weight in the back heel.

FOLLOW WITH:
prasarita padottanasana STANDING WIDE FORWARD BEND, PAGES 42–43
pindasana CHILD POSE, PAGES 20–21 AND
adho mukha svanasana DOWNWARD FACING DOG, PAGES 22–23

setu bandha sarvangasana

(BRIDGE POSE—HALF BACKARCH)

This half backarch is like a bridge spanning a river. The counterweights are on the near side in the head and shoulders; the supports are on the other side, in strong legs and feet. The breath makes an arc with the body from the back of the shoulders through the pelvis, down to the feet.

1 Start in Recuperation Pose I *(see page 26)*, arms by the sides, palms down. Exhale, letting the back of the waist touch the ground.

2 Let an in-breath come, exhale and, with the breath, raise the pelvis so that it arcs up. If the knees splay, tie a belt above them loosely, the same width as the hips. This keeps the weight in the feet, which are hip-width apart.

3 Breathe a full cycle of breath or more, then come down gently on the out-breath. Fold the knees into the chest, and rest. Repeat the pose twice.

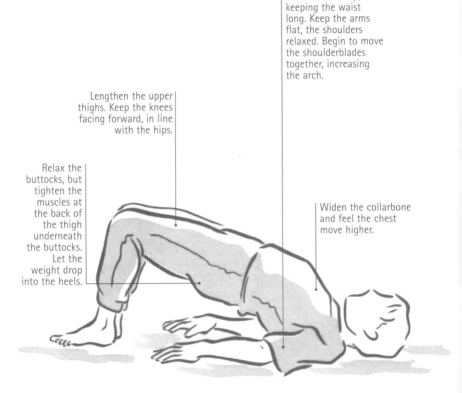

Arch the back up, keeping the waist long. Keep the arms flat, the shoulders relaxed. Begin to move the shoulderblades together, increasing the arch.

Lengthen the upper thighs. Keep the knees facing forward, in line with the hips.

Relax the buttocks, but tighten the muscles at the back of the thigh underneath the buttocks. Let the weight drop into the heels.

Widen the collarbone and feel the chest move higher.

jatara parivartanasana II

(SUPINE TWIST II)

A very useful twist, this is the next stage of the warming-up exercise on page 69, and benefits the shoulders and hips. The two-way turning of the spine is also very relaxing, helping calm body and mind, and encouraging sleep. When you first practice the pose, the two-way movement can be disorientating: Leave your head upright or watch the knees going down until you get used to it.

❶ Lie on your back and hug the knees in by holding them from beneath with the right arm.

❷ Place the left arm out to the side and look toward it.

❸ Exhale and roll the knees, the arm still holding them, to the right until the elbow comes to the ground.

❹ Remain in the pose, breathing until you feel relaxed. Come back to the center, and repeat on the other side. If the lower back is tense, bring yourself back to the center using the top leg.

The head looks toward the outstretched arm. The elbow rests on the floor with the arm beneath the thighs.

Keep the legs together, and relax the hips.

Relax the shoulders and roll the head away from the knees.

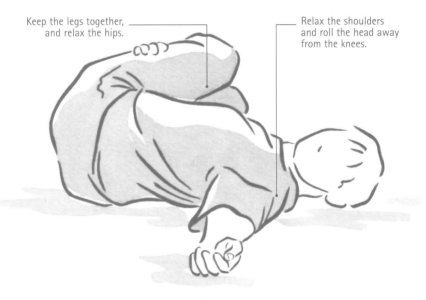

janu shirshasana

(SEATED HEAD-TO-KNEE)

Month 3 saw the open twisting version of this pose
(Parivrtta Janu Shirshasana, Twisting Head-to-Knee, pages
58–59), which you could include before or after this pose.
With one leg straight and one leg bent, Janu Shirshasana
is an easier forward bend for tight hamstrings. If one hip is
tighter, spend more time on that side. Work on a blanket.
If the bent knee is high, put cushions under the thigh.

❶ Sit on the floor, left leg straight and right leg bent to
the side, sole toward the left leg. Settle by taking the
hands behind, letting the legs relax, exhale and extend
upright.

❷ Exhale, feel the sitting bones, and lengthen up. On the
next exhalation, lengthen forward equally from each hip.

❸ Breathe as long as you feel the pose developing. If your
head touches the floor, continue lengthening on the out-
breath. Come up on an out-breath. Repeat on the other side.

Lengthen forward from both hips, keeping the spine centered. The shoulders and arms are relaxed, the chin in.

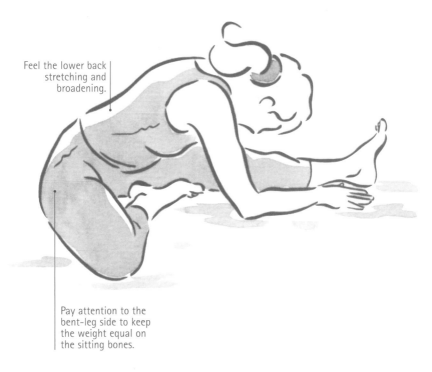

Feel the lower back stretching and broadening.

Pay attention to the bent-leg side to keep the weight equal on the sitting bones.

upavistha konasana

(OPEN ANGLE)

Like Pashchimottanasana (Seated Forward Bend, pages 46-47), this symmetrical pose is a soothing way to end a routine. It increases flexibility in the hips and lengthens the hamstrings.

The sitting bones, narrow and cushioned by the buttocks, are hard to visualize. They are like cups with a round base, and we tend to sit on the back of them. This exercise helps find the center of balance, with both sides of the cup vertical.

As with the first forward bend, those who are less flexible or have disk problems should bend forward onto a chair placed between the legs, folding the arms on the seat and resting the head on them. This lengthens the spine by relaxing the back of the legs and the sitting bones against the ground.

❶ Bend forward with legs apart. Feel heavy against the ground, "grounding" the body by making contact with and relaxing toward the floor.

❷ Breathe in the pose as long as is comfortable, lengthening on the out-breath and letting the in-breath come easily. Exhale to come back upright.

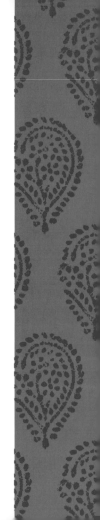

Toward the end of the exhalation, feel your abdominal muscles contract back toward the backbone. This protects the lower back by lengthening it down to the tailbone, and releases the upper back, allowing it to extend forward.

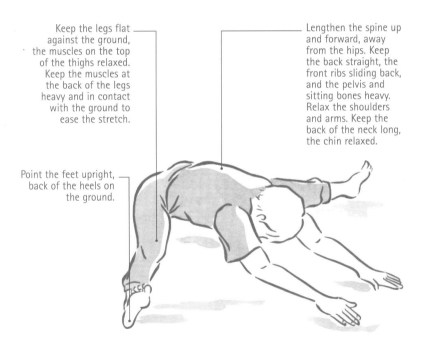

Keep the legs flat against the ground, the muscles on the top of the thighs relaxed. Keep the muscles at the back of the legs heavy and in contact with the ground to ease the stretch.

Lengthen the spine up and forward, away from the hips. Keep the back straight, the front ribs sliding back, and the pelvis and sitting bones heavy. Relax the shoulders and arms. Keep the back of the neck long, the chin relaxed.

Point the feet upright, back of the heels on the ground.

pranayama

Here, you add a pause or pauses to the breath. This is not holding the breath, rather a brief cessation in which nothing happens but stillness. In the stillness, the body weight drops down. The pause should not be longer than 3 seconds, and, to begin with, pause briefly, without strain. Never pause at the end of the out-breath: It will make you breathless.

❶ Sit or kneel comfortably, settle yourself, and start with the Ujjayi breath *(see page 25)*. When quiet, do a full cycle of breath and let the inhalation come freely.

❷ At the top of the inhalation, pause, exhale a little, pause, and exhale all the way. Let the in-breath come naturally, and repeat the pauses twice more, on the exhalation. Relax the shoulders and calm the face.

❸ Another day, repeat the cycle up to six times. Next time, increase the number of pauses on the exhalation to three, and repeat the cycle six times. Finally, lengthen the pauses to the count of 3, the intervals to the count of 2.

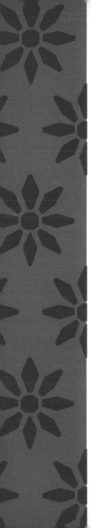

relaxation

However rushed you may be, always try to lie down for 5 to 10 minutes after your yoga practice. For some people, lying down can be an agony of impatience. The eyelids flutter, the eyes behind them moving from side to side; the hands are tense, and the fingers folded in. If this is you, try the exercise below. First settle in Recuperation Pose I *(see page 26)*. Cover the eyes with a hankerchief and place something heavy, a small stone, in the palm of each hand. When relaxed, lengthen the legs into Savasana *(see page 27)*. Exhale toward the back of the waist to relax it, and let the in-breath come naturally.

❶ Feel the imprint of your body against the ground. Relax the eyes behind closed eyelids, eyelashes resting gently on the cheeks. Lengthen the eyelids between the eyelashes and eyebrows.

❷ Keep the eyes quiet and look toward the hips. The face is calm, the backs of the hands heavy. After five cycles of conscious breathing, open the eyes, roll to one side, and get up slowly.

the story of yoga

Around 563 B.C.E., Siddhartha Gautama was born, a prince of the Shakyas, a small state on the border of modern Nepal. He grew up in prosperity and security. Although there was social upheaval in his land, there was also increased communication with countries as far away as Greece.

The story of Gautama tells that his father, the king, prevented his son from seeing the hardships of life by keeping him within the palace grounds. At 16, Gautama married and later had a son. When he was 29, he went outside the palace grounds for the first time and saw an old man, decrepit and leaning on a stick. He had not realized previously that old age afflicted men. Another time outside the grounds, he saw sickness, and a third time, he saw a corpse. Old age, sickness, and death became known as the "three marks of impermanence," and showed that life could not be divided from suffering. Siddhartha Gautama left his father's palace dressed humbly as a wandering ascetic, and began his search for enlightenment.

After studying with many gurus, Gautama came across a forest sect of naked monks who practiced severe austerities, believing pain and denial to be the source of release. Gautama argued that since it was through the mind that the body functioned, it was the mind that needed control, not the body.

When he was 35, Gautama arrived at Bodh Gaya, where he meditated beneath a banyan tree, swearing not to get up until he found enlightenment. After 49 days, during which he overcame many temptations, he attained Nirvana, the state of balance beyond the impermanence of ordinary life, and became the Buddha—the "Awakened One." He argued that since all existence was insubstantial, he had compassion for all beings caught in the endless cycle of suffering and rebirth, and understood the chain of actions that led to and caused suffering. With such experiences, he set out to become a teacher, and his teachings were collected by his disciples after his death in the Pali Canon.

The Buddha's teaching was rational and free from dogma, criticizing caste distinctions and the elite role of Brahmin priests, and his disciples grew numerous. He taught that enlightenment was by the Middle Way, a path between extremes, and through meditation, gave his followers practical ways to free themselves from the delusions of the ego-self. Nirvana was available to all who followed the Eight-fold Path, which comprized right understanding, right intention, right speech, right action, right livelihood, right effort, right awareness, and right concentration (samadhi).

As Buddhism developed, it changed into different forms and established itself as a world religion, although it faded in popularity in India with the rise of Hinduism.

month5

Celebrate midsummer, time of picnics and lazing on the sand, with a feast of yoga poses to benefit the hips and knees. The seated Hero Poses help the hips become more flexible for kneeling and sitting, the Twisting Triangle relaxes the knees while keeping the shoulders supple, and the month's yoga sequence finishes with the famous Cobbler's Pose. The subject of the month is kneeling and stretching—natural movements that make everyday actions easier. Breathing focuses on the body's two inner channels of energy, with alternate-nostril breathing to balance the left- and right-hand sides of the body.

key postures:

warming up (RECLINING BOUND—ANGLE POSE)

salabhasana (LOCUST POSE)

virasana (HERO POSE)

parivrtta trikonasana (TWISTING TRIANGLE)

ardha mandalasana (LUNGE POSE)

supta baddha konasana (COBBLER'S POSE)

pranayama (ALTERNATE—NOSTRIL BREATHING)

relaxation

kneeling and stretching

Sitting on chairs, driving, and repetitive work all tighten the hips and shoulders. You can start to counter such restrictive ways of moving by taking time to sit on the ground at a picnic this summer, or walk on grass, which, unlike hard sidewalks that compress the hips and knees, promotes natural movement.

Yoga also restores to the body movements that should be instinctive, making everyday actions easier. Having greater consciousness of the feet puts a spring back in your step. Straightening your knees and being conscious of your center of gravity helps with waiting and standing. Kneeling is something else we do everyday without thinking, whether kneeling to play with a child or work in the garden, and benefits from the awareness yoga brings to it.

The knee joint is a sophisticated structure bound together with strong ligaments. Rigorous exercise is not the way to loosen the knees; the best way to exercise them is to work the hips above and the feet below. The knee is relaxed when straight, so yoga poses with straight legs are a real help for stiff knees. If you feel pressure in the knee when kneeling, your center of gravity is too far forward. Use the kneeling Hero Poses *(see pages 96-99)* to warm the hips and take the center of gravity back, allowing the body to stretch forward more easily.

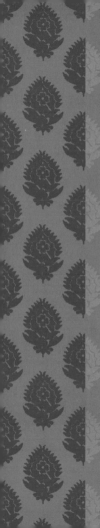

warming up

Start your session by yawning. Open your mouth, let in the in-breath, and you will soon find yourself yawning, releasing the jaw and neck. Practice the supine leg stretches on pages 34-35, Lying Down Diamond *(see page 51)*, and Supine Twist I *(see page 69)*, then the pose below.

supta baddha konasana

(RECLINING BOUND—ANGLE POSE)

❶ Lie on your back and place the soles of the feet together, with the sides of the feet resting on the ground a comfortable distance in front of the tailbone.

❷ Exhale and drop the knees down and out to either side.

❸ Feel the spine against the ground and the long back of the waist. As you exhale, be conscious of the whole inner length of the spine. If the ligaments across the groin feel tight, press the soles together to release them. Or bring the knees up and, exhaling, drop them gradually out again, soles together. Hold as long as is comfortable.

salabhasana (LOCUST POSE)

This subtle backbend strengthens the muscles in the lower back. Keep the back of the waist long and lengthen forward while coming up so as not to compress the lower back. Let a full in-breath come before moving on the out-breath. Do only three or four, including variations.

❶ LOCUST STAGE 1 Lie on your front, arms to either side, palms up. Rest the forehead on the ground, keeping the back of the neck long.

❷ Exhale toward the back of the waist and let the upper body lengthen forward and up. Keep the chin in. Bring the arms up behind, palms facing each other.

❸ Take a full cycle of breath, if possible, lengthening on the out-breath, before relaxing down. Rest before repeating the pose, using the arm variations below, if desired.

❹ LOCUST STAGE 2 Clasp the hands behind the skull, elbows out. LOCUST STAGE 3 Stretch the arms out in front and rise up from the ground as the torso lengthens forward and up.

(LOCUST POSE)

Always do a forward bend like Balasana (CHILD POSE) after backbends.

Keep the pelvis heavy, the pubic bone and legs down, buttocks relaxed. The tailbone lengthens downward.

Lengthen the back of the waist. Take the shoulders down and back as the arms come up, palms facing. Keep the back of the neck long, chin in.

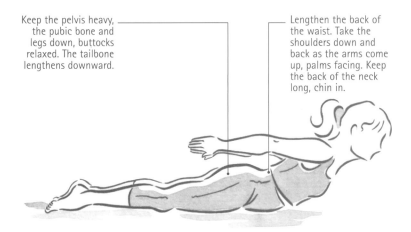

FOLLOW WITH:
balasana CHILD POSE, PAGES 20-21
eka pada rajakapotasana
ONE LEGGED PIGEON POSE I, PAGES 54-55

virasana (HERO POSE)

Hero Pose is good for the hips and takes the center of gravity back by dropping the body weight into the sitting bones. It also stretches the top of the thighs and works the feet.

 The hips and the tops of the feet need to be flexible for this pose. If you feel knee strain or are uncomfortable, place cushions under your buttocks and a rolled-up blanket under the top of the feet. If the knees feel strained with the cushions, omit Hero Pose, and continue the rest of the routine.

1 Kneel and sit between your feet, thighs turned inward.

2 HERO STAGE 1 Breathe, exhaling and letting the sitting bones drop. Take time before moving to the next stages.

3 HERO STAGE 2 With hands on soles, leave the pelvis down, exhale and bend forward *(see illustration, page 98)*. Come up.

4 HERO STAGE 3 Place the hands down behind, and breathe the body back, elbows bent, tail curving under. Lie flat back, if able *(see illustration, page 98)*. Come up; sit straight legged.

(HERO POSE, STAGE 1)

Take time, with lots of breathing to settle into these Hero Poses. Sitting on cushions helps the muscles to relax and can be taken away as you become more flexible.

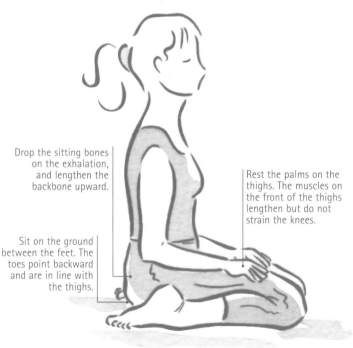

Drop the sitting bones on the exhalation, and lengthen the backbone upward.

Rest the palms on the thighs. The muscles on the front of the thighs lengthen but do not strain the knees.

Sit on the ground between the feet. The toes point backward and are in line with the thighs.

virasana

(HERO POSE, STAGE 2)

Place the hands on the soles of the feet. Leave the pelvis on the ground, breathe out, and bend forward.

With each out-breath, lengthen the lower back. When you can no longer go forward and keep the hips on the ground, let the tail come up.

Put your forehead on the ground. Breathe back to the hips, letting the pelvis drop, before returning upright.

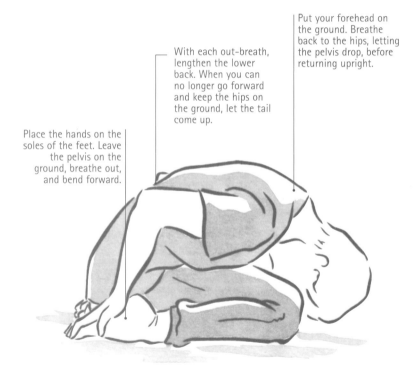

(HERO POSE, STAGE 3)

When you reach the floor after extending back, lie flat and lengthen the back of the waist, using cushions beneath the lower back and shoulders, if necessary.

As you go back, do not overcurve the back of the waist: Lengthen it, and focus on curving the tailbone under the pelvis, as if it would extend along the floor between the knees.

Keep the knees together and down, but not over-strained. Lengthen the muscles on the front of the thighs. It may help to let the knees come up, relax, and drop again.

FOLLOW WITH:

tadasana MOUNTAIN POSE, PAGES 14–15
virabhadrasana WARRIOR POSE, PAGES 60–61
uttanasana STANDING FORWARD BEND, PAGE 19
trikonasana TRIANGLE POSE, PAGES 71–73

parivrtta trikonasana

(TWISTING TRIANGLE)

Whereas in Trikonasana (Triangle Pose, pages 71-73), the body extended sideways when going forward, this version reverses the turn. It is slightly harder, and you experience the extension more by taking a longer step forward.

❶ From Tadasana *(see pages 14-15)*, take the weight onto the left leg and with the right, take a longer step forward than in Trikonasana *(see page 71)*. The weight stays in the back heel, although there is more weight on the front foot.

❷ Exhale, turning to the right, and extend the right arm behind, looking toward it. Breathe, grounding the back heel and turning.

❸ Exhale and extend the turned body forward and down, the right arm extending up.

❹ Breathe, developing the pose, exhale, and come back upright. Repeat on the other side.

Remember that as the back heel is down, it will limit the amount your body can go forward.

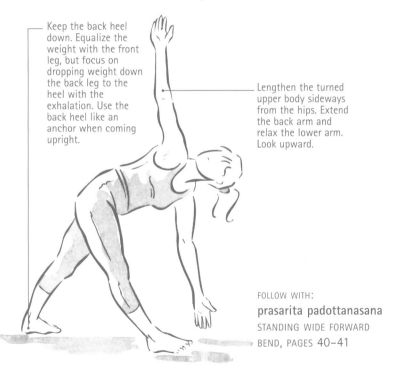

Keep the back heel down. Equalize the weight with the front leg, but focus on dropping weight down the back leg to the heel with the exhalation. Use the back heel like an anchor when coming upright.

Lengthen the turned upper body sideways from the hips. Extend the back arm and relax the lower arm. Look upward.

FOLLOW WITH:
prasarita padottanasana
STANDING WIDE FORWARD
BEND, PAGES 40–41

ardha mandalasana

(LUNGE POSE)

This asana lengthens the lower back easily, and works the hip over the bent knee. The main weight of the pose stays in the front heel, the foot flat and strong against the ground. It is from this side that the hip sinks down, not where the long leg stretches away. The back leg releases from hip to knee, but does not over-stretch the front of the groin, which is delicate. You can also get into the pose by stepping back from Uttanasana *(see page 19).*

❶ From hands and knees, bring the right leg forward and place the foot flat, heel down.

❷ Take the left leg back, the knee resting on the ground, the toes curled under.

❸ Exhale toward the back of the waist, bringing the torso up, and lengthening from the crown of the head to the back heel. As the in-breath comes, feel the back ribs widen. Hold as long as is comfortable, and repeat on the other side.

Keep the hips level, the weight dropping more into the hip of the bent leg. Do not sag into or overstretch the front of the thigh of the long leg.

Lengthen the back of the neck, chin in.

Place the knee over the foot.

Curl the toes under, and extend the heel.

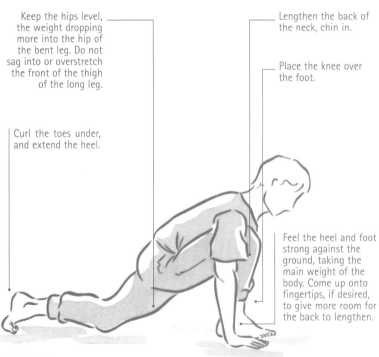

Feel the heel and foot strong against the ground, taking the main weight of the body. Come up onto fingertips, if desired, to give more room for the back to lengthen.

FOLLOW WITH:
balasana AND **adho mukha svanasana sequence** CHILD POSE AND DOWNWARD FACING DOG, PAGE 20–23

baddha konasana

(COBBLER'S POSE)

As the name suggests, cobblers used this position while working, the shoe placed upright between the feet so the sole could be sewn easily. It is one of the oldest yoga poses, pictured on seals discovered in the Indus Valley from the Harappa civilization that flourished around 2500 B.C.E. Baddha Konasana can be used during pranayama, but, for many of us, the thighs stay too high to be truly comfortable. Practice frequently to help the thighs drop down.

❶ From sitting, bend the knees out and bring the soles of the feet together. With your hands, massage the soles, turning them upward.

❷ Sit tall and breathe, feeling the sitting bones beneath you. Relax the knees.

❸ Exhale and lengthen forward. Keep the hands where they are, opening the feet, or place them in front on the ground. Stay in the pose as long as is comfortable.

Opening the soles of the feet lowers the knees as the thighs turn outward. Let the pose develop rather than forcing it, staying more upright until the thighs release down. While upright, keep the shoulders relaxed and wide, the back of the neck long and the chin in. Exhale toward the back of the waist, the weight in the sitting bones, and lengthen upward.

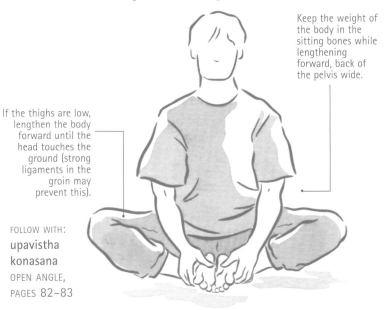

Keep the weight of the body in the sitting bones while lengthening forward, back of the pelvis wide.

If the thighs are low, lengthen the body forward until the head touches the ground (strong ligaments in the groin may prevent this).

FOLLOW WITH:
upavistha konasana
OPEN ANGLE,
PAGES 82–83

pranayama

(NADI SODHANA—ALTERNATE-NOSTRIL BREATHING)

Hatha yoga holds that two channels of energy spiral around the spine and relate to the breath from each nostril: *Ida*, the moon (left) channel; and *pingala*, the sun (right) channel.

❶ Sit or kneel, using the Ujjayi breath *(see page 25)*.

❷ Exert light pressure on the bony side of the nose, above the nostril flare. To begin, use the tip of the index finger. To use the whole (right) hand, put the knuckles of the index and middle fingers above the bridge of the nose between the eyes. Ring and little fingers block the left nostril, thumb the right.

❸ Let an in-breath come. Block the left nostril; exhale, then inhale through the right. Then block the right nostril; exhale and inhale through the left. Continue for several cycles, as is comfortable.

❹ To end: Exhale through the right nostril, inhale through both. Do three to five cycles on each side.

relaxation

Finish this month's routine with at least five cycles of Ujjayi breathing *(see page 24)* before lying in Recuperation Pose I *(see page 26)*. Make yourself warm and comfortable, and relax against the ground. When you feel stable and quiet, lengthen the legs into Savasana *(see page 27)*. Relax, breathing the back of the waist long, and feel the back of the legs heavy. Relax the shoulders and hips. Feel the floor against the back of the body and relax further against it.

❶ Feel the out-breath start at the back of the throat, dropping behind the collarbone, down behind the front ribs, and behind the stomach. Let the body remain passive as the in-breath enters, widening the sides and back ribs.

❷ Relax the jaw, the eyes, and the forehead. Feel the wide space between the ears at the back of the head. Exhale to the outer edges of the body, and observe the in-breath.

❸ After five cycles of conscious breathing, open the eyes, roll to one side, stretch, and finally, get up slowly.

the story of yoga

Jainism pre-dates and was contemporary with the lifetime of the Buddha. It was founded by Mahavira (c.599–527 B.C.E.), the last of 24 Fordmakers—fabled teachers who had attained wisdom by renouncing the material world.

Mahavira, like the Buddha, came from the warrior estate in northeast India. He rejected the caste system and the authority of the Brahmin priests, and sought to transcend the cycle of birth and death through rigorous asceticism. He preached that through the practice of renunciation (right faith, right knowledge, and right conduct), the soul could be freed from karma. A further code included five vows: Not to kill, speak untruth, nor steal; continence (being chaste); and the renunciation of pleasure in the external. Mahatma Gandhi (1869–1948), the leading force behind modern India's independence, came from Gujurat, the center of Jainism from the 3rd century A.D., and was influenced by the doctrine of non-violence, which he used in his civil-rights campaigns.

Jaina non-violence was present in every aspect of life. As all life forms were thought to have a soul (jiva) that seeks release, Jains to this day are strictly vegetarian, abstaining also from fruits with many seeds and fermented drinks.

Yoga in Jainism was the way to transcend the effects of karma through meditation. Later Jaina writers detail specific postures: Vajrasana (see page 52), Sukhasana (see sitting cross legged, page 24), and Padmasana Lotus (see page 244).

Around 327–325 B.C.E., Alexander the Great briefly invaded northern India, and in 321, a new leader, Chandragupta, usurped the Maghada throne and founded the Maurya Dynasty, establishing a state from the Indus to the Ganges and north into Afghanistan. His last days were spent, reputedly, with Jains in a Mysore retreat, ritually starving himself to death.

Chandragupta's descendants expanded the Maurya empire to the south until the whole of India came under political unity with Asoka (c.269–232 B.C.E.). Literacy increased, and the state boasted an army, tax system, and bureaucracy. Asoka converted to Buddhism after an horrific battle. He expressed his Buddhism in a series of inscriptions. These requested respect for the dignity of all peoples, religious toleration, and practice of non-violence. He also decreed that banyan trees should be planted along roads to provide shade. However, these idealistic measures did not impress the majority of Indians, and there were sectarian struggles and suspicion from the Brahmin priests.

The assault on the Brahmanical religion from disaffected sects and the threat of Asoka's Buddhism led to a ferment of thought illustrated in and influenced by the Upanishadic writings. From this, early Hinduism developed.

month 6

In the lazy days of high summer it can be difficult to keep up the enthusiasm for diligent yoga practice. In this month's sequences, poses to inspire and keep the spirits lifted include Sage Pose, and, appropriately, the theme for the month is studying and growing. Further seated and twisting asanas also stretch the body to make sitting easier. This month's breathing exercise introduces Kapalabhati, a cleansing and rejuvenating treatment for the lungs.

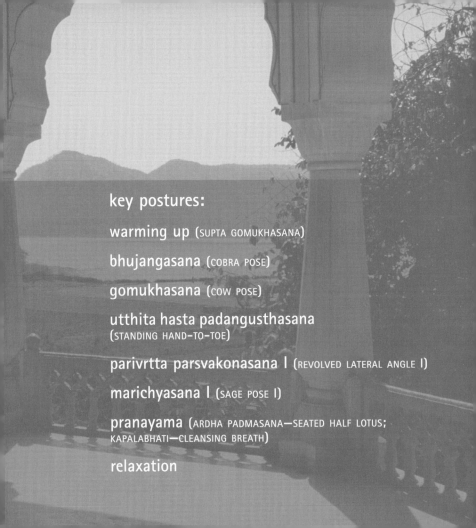

studying and growing

Yoga is a physical and mental discipline, which helps to establish the balance, stability, and resources that mind and body need to function smoothly. This in turn frees up your mind, body, and spirit to develop their true potential. The path to growth is not always smooth and can take you to unexpected places. This tale is revealing: A soccer player, after taking up yoga, found his physical ability to play improved to legendary heights. However, one day, when the moment came for the match to be won, the player found he no longer needed to win and had lost the competitive ruthlessness required to score. Even though the crowds were disappointed, the player had grown in understanding.

The path to practicing is also not smooth. After the first burst of enthusiasm, it's easy to fall out of the habit. A week without yoga becomes two weeks, then we start to wonder if it's worth practicing at all. When facing illness or crisis, we return to yoga, but how much better if it had been there all the time.

Try to approach yoga practice without expectation, and don't let the days when nothing goes right block memories of the good times. The benefits of practice are great. Listen to the body and be sensitive to its demands, and see how your body responds and your mind clears of doubts. Yoga is a tool that helps every part of life.

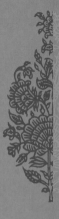

warming up

Start in Recuperation Pose II *(see page 33)*. Focus on the breath, and feel the exhalation undoing tensions. Follow with the supine leg stretches on pages 34–35. Add Supta Baddha Konasana *(see page 91)* before the pose below, which warms the hips.

supta gomukhasana
(COW LEGS)

❶ Lying on your back, bend the knees and place the right knee over the left knee.

❷ Fold crossed knees in toward the chest, hands beneath the thighs. Exhale toward tight areas, working and releasing them.

❸ To increase the stretch, place the left hand on the top shin, the right hand on the lower shin, and take the legs apart slightly. Repeat with the left leg crossed over the right.

bhujangasana

(COBRA POSE)

In Hindu mythology, the snake has the opposing attributes of destroyer and protector, and this pose resembles a serpent or cobra about to strike. As in Salabhasana (Locust Pose, pages 94–95), which you should practice first, the torso comes up as the spine lengthens forward and up. The shoulders stay relaxed and weight drops into the hands. Repeat the pose three times, resting between.

❶ Lie on your stomach, hands underneath the shoulders, elbows bent. Exhale, and practice lengthening the back of the waist to the tailbone. Keep buttocks and legs relaxed.

❷ Inhale and then, as you exhale, lengthen the torso forward and up, the weight dropping into the hands. Tuck in the chin so the back of the neck and head are long and broad like the hood of the cobra.

❸ Straighten the elbows, but do not compress the lower back. Be patient: Don't push up too far too soon, and do not stay in the pose long. Exhale and come down; rest.

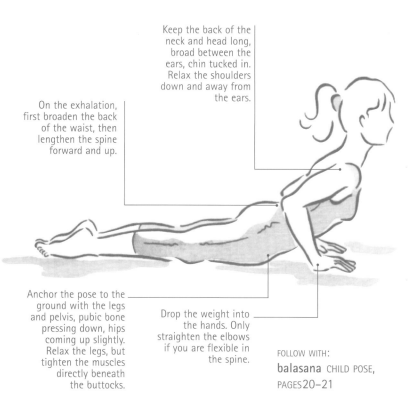

Keep the back of the neck and head long, broad between the ears, chin tucked in. Relax the shoulders down and away from the ears.

On the exhalation, first broaden the back of the waist, then lengthen the spine forward and up.

Anchor the pose to the ground with the legs and pelvis, pubic bone pressing down, hips coming up slightly. Relax the legs, but tighten the muscles directly beneath the buttocks.

Drop the weight into the hands. Only straighten the elbows if you are flexible in the spine.

FOLLOW WITH:
balasana CHILD POSE,
PAGES 20–21

gomukhasana
(COW POSE)

Here is the full Cow Pose to benefit the shoulders and
outside of the hips, and make the leg muscles more
elastic. The pose resembles a cow's face, broad at one end
and narrow at the other. In Hindu mythology, the cow
represents fertility and abundance.

1 From sitting, fold in the right leg so the side of the
thigh is on the ground, the knee centered as far as possible
in front. The side of the foot stays on the ground.

2 Bend the left leg, taking the left foot over the right
knee toward the right hip. Ideally, the knees should be on
top of each other, but, to begin with, it is more important
that both sitting bones stay down.

3 Sit upright, breathe the sitting bones down, and lengthen
the spine. When ready, add the Cow Arms on page 70, then
the Eagle Arms on page 37. Repeat on the other side.

Start this pose with the legs only and then add the arms.

On the exhalation, relax the hips, feeling the weight in the sitting bones. Let the Cow Arms straighten the back and the exhalation lengthen the spine upward.

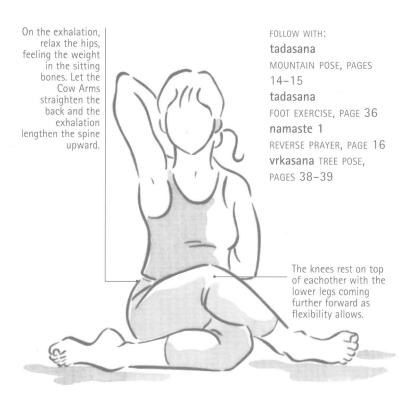

FOLLOW WITH:

tadasana
MOUNTAIN POSE, PAGES 14–15

tadasana
FOOT EXERCISE, PAGE 36

namaste 1
REVERSE PRAYER, PAGE 16

vrkasana TREE POSE, PAGES 38–39

The knees rest on top of eachother with the lower legs coming further forward as flexibility allows.

utthita hasta padangusthasana
(STANDING HAND-TO-TOE)

Try this balance to strengthen the legs, and lend poise
and steadiness to the body. Make sure, both when hugging
the leg in and extending it, that the hip on the same side
drops down. This creates less disturbance to the weight
over the standing leg and also lengthens the lower back.

❶ Stand in Tadasana *(see pages 14–15)* and take the
weight onto the left leg.

❷ Bend the right knee up and hug it in toward the chest,
hands under or over the knee.

❸ Catch the foot in the right hand, or with a belt *(see
illustration on page 117)*, and, as you exhale, extend the
leg forward. Once the leg is straight, move it upward on
each out-breath. Maintain a straight back. Hold the pose
as long as comfort allows. Repeat on the other side.

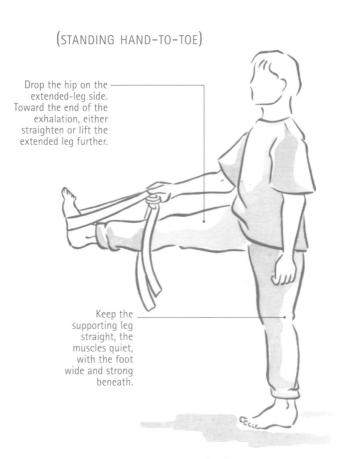

(STANDING HAND-TO-TOE)

Drop the hip on the extended-leg side. Toward the end of the exhalation, either straighten or lift the extended leg further.

Keep the supporting leg straight, the muscles quiet, with the foot wide and strong beneath.

parivrtta parsvakonasana I

(REVOLVED LATERAL ANGLE I)

This twist starts from Ardha Mandalasana *(see pages 100–101)*. Move into it from the forward bend Uttanasana *(see page 19)*. If your hands touch the ground in Uttanasana, take a long step back with the right leg, knee on the ground, toes curled under. If the hands don't yet reach the ground, bend the knees and step back. Practice a few times on each side.

❶ From Ardha Mandalasana, bend forward, place the hands to either side of the left foot, and relax the hips. Move the left hand to the floor inside the left knee.

❷ Exhale, turning the shoulders and body to the right and up. Bring the left hand onto fingertips (a long arm helps the turn). Place the right hand behind the waist and look up.

❸ To extend the twist, exhale, stretch the right heel away, and straighten the right leg. On another exhalation, take the right arm over the head. Hold, developing stability in the front heel and the line of the body. Repeat on the other side.

FOLLOW WITH:

balasana AND **adho
mukha svanasana
sequence** CHILD POSE AND
DOWNWARD FACING DOG,
PAGES 20-23
**setu bandha
sarvangasana** BRIDGE
POSE–HALF BACKARCH,
PAGES 76-77
jatara parivartanasana II
SUPINE TWIST II, PAGES
78-79

Take the arm over the
head, or behind the
waist to begin with,
if you prefer.

Exhale toward the back
of the waist to help
the turn and improve
the line from the crown
of the head or top
hand to the back heel.

Keep the feet facing
forward, the main
weight in the front
heel. Open the body
outward and
straighten the
back leg.

marichyasana I

(SAGE POSE I)

It is a wise person that can turn all ways, and this asana
is named after the sage Marichi. The twist here is a more
advanced pose that shouldn't be forced. If you prefer, ease
the pose with a more open twist: Come upright after step
1, turn away from the knee, and place the back hand down
behind, leaving the front arm extended inside the bent knee.

❶ Sit with the the right leg straight, the left knee bent
up. Exhale and sit up straight. On another exhalation,
bend forward, and place the left arm inside the left thigh.

❷ Keep extending forward. When the left shoulder is
below the knee, wrap the arm back around the knee.

❸ Exhale, turning the body to the right. Take the right
arm around the back of the waist and catch the left hand.
If the hands do not connect, use a belt.

❹ Exhale upright, turn into the twist, and look over the
right shoulder. Hold, developing the twist. Repeat to the left.

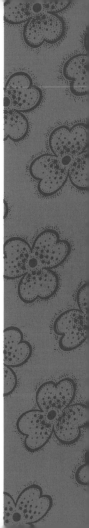

Keep the weight in both sitting bones and use the exhalation to help the torso turn. Let the in-breath come easily.

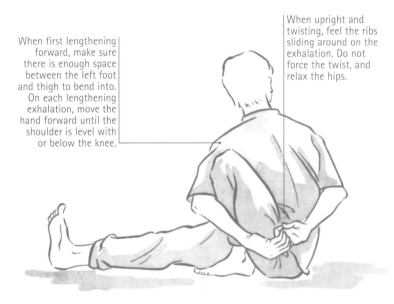

When upright and twisting, feel the ribs sliding around on the exhalation. Do not force the twist, and relax the hips.

When first lengthening forward, make sure there is enough space between the left foot and thigh to bend into. On each lengthening exhalation, move the hand forward until the shoulder is level with or below the knee.

FOLLOW WITH:
paschimottanasana SITTING FORWARD BEND, PAGES 42-43

pranayama

(ARDHA PADMASANA—SEATED HALF LOTUS)

For this month's breathing, try sitting in Half Lotus position.

❶ From sitting cross-legged, take the left foot, left hand behind the ankle, the right hand behind the toes, and draw it into the hip of the opposite leg, resting it on the thigh. Turn the left thigh outward to help the rotation in the hip. Relax the knee and thigh with no strain in the knee.

❷ Sit with one leg on top for one day's breathing, and the other leg uppermost the next day. If you don't find the pose comfortable, return to sitting cross-legged, but vary which leg rests on top with each breathing session.

kapalabhati
(CLEANSING BREATH)

This breathing technique is like shaking the feathers in a pillow down to one end. It cleanses the lungs with a series of short abdominal contractions on the exhalation of breath. These are like soft punches to the stomach that expel air, massaging the internal organs and toning the abdominal muscles.

On the exhalation, the abdomen is pulled in sharply, and then releases in an action similar to sneezing. As the abdomen contracts, it expels air; and as it releases, a small amount of oxygen enters the lungs, allowing many contractions and releases to be sustained over one exhalation.

Kapalabhati cleans stale air out of the lungs and is an excellent preparation for other breathing exercises. Therefore, in different breathing sessions, follow Kapalabhati and Ujjayi breathing *(see page 25)* with either Viloma on the out-breath *(see page 84)* or Nadi Sodhana, alternate-nostril breathing *(see page 104)*.

Cautions: Seek medical advice before practicing Kapalabhati if you have heart or lung problems, high blood pressure, or eye or ear disorders. Avoid if you are pregnant or suffering from prolapse. If you feel lightheaded or hyperventilate, stop immediately: You are not practicing Kapalabhati correctly or have performed too many.

kapalabhati (CLEANSING BREATH)

❶ Sit straight. Lengthen the back of the waist, hips relaxed. Breathing through the nose, let the in-breath come.

❷ At the top of the in-breath, with lungs full, contract the abdomen sharply, forcing the air out, then relax it. Exhale the rest of the air; let the in-breath come naturally.

❸ Breathe a full cycle of regular exhalation and inhalation. At the top of the inhalation, repeat the contraction and release of the abdomen, repeat a second time, then exhale the rest of the air. Let the in-breath come naturally.

❹ After a cycle of regular breathing, repeat a third time. To begin with, try only two or three Kapalabhati on the exhalation, with a full cycle of regular breathing between. Repeat or increase the number on the next exhalation. After practice, increase the number of Kapalabhatis on the exhalation, always taking a full cycle of regular breathing between, and repeating only three times. Work up to 20 or 30 Kapalabhati on an exhalation: Return to Ujjayi breathing before practicing a different breathing variation.

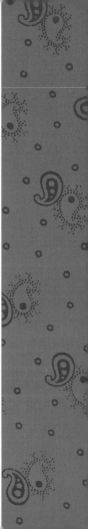

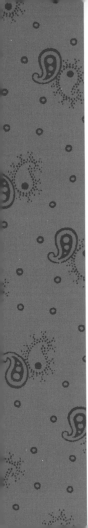

relaxation

Finish pranayama with regular Ujjayi breathing *(see page 25)*, and lie in Recuperation Pose I *(see page 26)*. Let your breath quiet, and then use the Ujjayi breath to ground the back of the body. Exhale, using the inside of the spine as the path for the breath and contracting the abdomen toward the end. As the abdomen relaxes, receive the in-breath passively. Lengthen the legs into Savasana *(see page 27)*. Exhale toward the back of the waist to lengthen it, and relax the hips and legs.

❶ Relax the shoulders, feeling more of the ground beneath them. Feel the backs of the hands heavy against the floor. The palms are open, the skin soft, the air passing over them.

❷ Relax the face and lengthen the back of the neck. Relax the throat and feel the out-breath as it moves down the back of the throat and travels down the body. Observe the in-breath entering the body.

❸ After five cycles of conscious breathing, open the eyes, roll to one side, and get up slowly.

the story of yoga

In early Hinduism, the Vedic gods became more fixed in a central trimurti of Brahma, abstract creator of the universe; Vishnu, the Preserver; and Shiva, the Destroyer and Lord of Yoga because of his practice of austerities and meditation. Vishnu, a solar deity, fought on the side of good and came down to earth to help mankind—two of his most famous human incarnations were Rama and Krishna. Of uncertain dates in the 2nd and 3rd centuries B.C.E., two remarkable epic poems helped popularize religious teachings for a wider audience: The Ramayana and the Mahabharata. Both contain extraordinary tales of love, honor, and war, and their inclusion of incarnations (avatars) of a god in human form acting as an intermediary between mortals and the divine, made religion more approachable. The epics also contributed to a moral code of conduct: Their mythical characters, complete with human weaknesses, were readily identified with.

Comprising 24,000 verses, the Ramayana begins in the country of Koshala, where aged king Dasharatha has stated that his son, Rama, will ucceed him. One of Dasharatha's three wives, to whom he owes two boons, asks for her own son, Bharata, to be appointed, and for Rama to be exiled for 14 years. Unable to refuse, Dasharatha banishes Rama, who, with unquestioning filial obedience, retires to the forest with his wife Sita. On the death of the king, Bharata refuses the throne and goes to look for his half-brother. Rama, honoring his banishment, refuses to return and battles the demons of the forest, who were terrifying its people. The greatest demon, Ravana, kidnaps Sita and takes her to Lanka. For many years Rama searches for her until, with the help of the monkey king, Hanuman, he kills Ravana and rescues Sita. Although Sita pleads her innocence, Rama assumes his wife has been defiled by the demon, and banishes her. Sita insists that Rama let the Divine decide her fate and, entering a burning pyre, is untouched by the flames. Rama repents and is reunited with his wife. The couple return to the capital to rule with Bharata in a just and ideal regime.

Rama is the personification of the righteous hero despite his suspicion of Sita, who symbolizes chastity and kindness. Hanuman, the monkey hero, is Rama's most devoted follower, and the personification of devotion (bhakti) yoga. For selflessly sorting out the problems of the heroic couple, Hanuman was worshiped in his turn. In the 14th century A.D., the guru Ramananda returned the development of bhakti yoga from southern India to northern India, and Hanuman became one of its principle deities. His name is given to a yoga asana commemorating his great leap to fetch a healing herb for the fatally injured Rama. Similar to the gymnastic splits, the pose is an extension of Eka Pada Rajakapotasana (see pages 54–55).

In the Ramayana, Rama demonstrates self-discipline, moral vigor, and equanimity, and symbolizes moral virtues: Observances (yama) and restraints (niyama) codified later by Pantanjali in the classical exposition of yoga.

section II index

ripening

The blush of summer's ripening and the move into fall brings you to more advanced yoga poses. Move through these months in sequence, getting to know each asana before moving onto the next. Do not measure success in how well you perform a pose, but in how much you learn about your body and yourself. The inverted asanas can take time to feel familiar, but the preparation toward them is of great benefit. Intersperse routines from the previous six months, as desired.

month 7
month 8
month 9

month 7

There is an inner strength and centeredness in the poses offered in the first of this season's yoga sequences. Crane Pose is a hand balance, the crane a marsh bird that stands silently at the edge of water. Preparation begins for inversions, perhaps the most deeply calming and mentally beneficial of all the yoga asanas. The month's topic for thought is the intense power of squatting and reaching out, while fall's first breathing exercise counters the heat of the physical exertion, as well as of the season, with Sitali, a cooling breath.

key postures:

warming up (SUPTA ARDHA PADMASANA)

ushtrasana (CAMEL POSE)

garudasana (EAGLE POSE)

malasana (GARLAND POSE)

bakasana (CRANE POSE)

sarvangasana (SHOULDER STAND—STAGE 1)

parivrtta upavistha konasana (TWISTING SEATED ANGLE)

pranayama (SITALI—COOLING BREATH)

relaxation

squatting and reaching

Yoga can give us powers we did not seem to have before. These are an expression of joy from a body growing supple and stronger. There are many stories of powers performed by yogis: Levitation, walking across burning coals, becoming invisible, or holding the breath for days or months. These are mystical and misty apparitions. Yoga is not about acquiring these powers, nor is it for show. A strong desire to demonstrate what you have achieved is natural, but not necessary: What you are doing shows in your health, in the way you hold yourself, and in the happier, more concentrated state of your mind. There is always more to discover.

Squatting is a working pose for field hands and gardeners, and a natural movement for toddlers. From the strong base of the feet, the body reaches forward so that the hands touch the ground. To begin with, it may seem as though you have no power left to reach out. With perseverance, power is learned again.

The squatting poses in the sequence that follows are intense forward bends that use muscles deep in the abdomen. They offer a feeling of inner strength and also of centeredness, which is of absolute necessity when taking the body into the hand balance. They are powerful poses, but the process of doing them can be humbling. One can literally fall over backward or sprawl out forward.

warming up

Start with the supine leg stretches on pages 34–35, then practice Supta Gomukhasana (Cow Legs, page 111).

supta ardha padmasana
(LYING DOWN HALF LOTUS)

Here, the hip rotates as the thigh turns out, with no strain in the knee. If you do feel strain, don't draw the foot higher.

❶ From Recuperation Pose II *(see page 33)*, bend in the right leg and hold the foot, right hand under the ankle, left hand under the toes, knee out to the side.

❷ Draw the foot up the left thigh and rest it in the fold of the hip. Release the right hand.

❸ Exhale; straighten the left leg, taking the right knee down too. Hold the right foot, sole upward, lightly behind the toes with the left hand or a belt, shoulders straight.

❹ Exhale and relax the right knee. Repeat on other leg.

ushtrasana

(CAMEL POSE)

The arch of the body here resembles a camel's hump. The key to the pose is the lengthening of the spine, and it is an excellent way to encourage this in the upper back. Using the upper back lifts pressure from the back of the waist, where the muscles also have to lengthen to avoid constriction. If the back of the waist feels uncomfortable, return upright and bend forward before trying again. Starting with the hands in Inverted Prayer *(see page 16)* can help the upper back to move. As you go further back, drop the hands to the heels.

❶ With knees on the ground, body vertical above, relax the thighs. Exhale, and lengthen up.

❷ When you can grow no taller, exhale and begin to lengthen backward. Drop the arms behind until the hands catch the heels.

❸ Hold briefly, and come up. Kneel forward and rest. Repeat the pose, then kneel forward for at least 10 breath cycles.

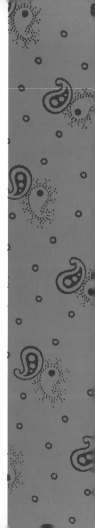

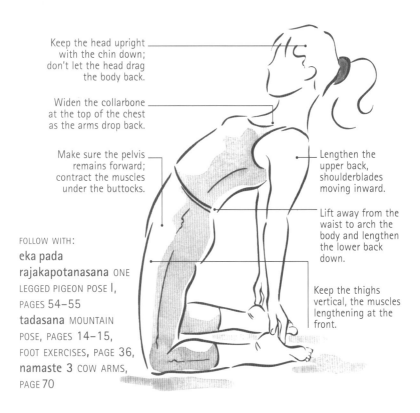

Keep the head upright with the chin down; don't let the head drag the body back.

Widen the collarbone at the top of the chest as the arms drop back.

Make sure the pelvis remains forward; contract the muscles under the buttocks.

Lengthen the upper back, shoulderblades moving inward.

Lift away from the waist to arch the body and lengthen the lower back down.

Keep the thighs vertical, the muscles lengthening at the front.

FOLLOW WITH:
eka pada rajakapotanasana ONE LEGGED PIGEON POSE I, PAGES 54–55
tadasana MOUNTAIN POSE, PAGES 14–15, FOOT EXERCISES, PAGE 36, **namaste 3** COW ARMS, PAGE 70

garudasana

(EAGLE POSE)

This balancing pose is named after the eagle Garuda, in Hindu mythology, the immortal bird ridden by Vishnu, Lord of the Universe. It broadens the back of the pelvis, and establishes firmness in the heel of the supporting leg.

1 From Tadasana *(see pages 14–15)*, take the weight onto the right leg and bend the knee, leaving the heel down.

2 Cross the left leg over the knee and wrap the lower leg around the right calf, toes hooked around the shin.

3 Exhale and move the arms into Eagle Arms *(see page 37)*, either the opposite way or the same way as the legs. Remember which way the arms are crossed.

4 Exhale and lengthen upward. Relax the hips, and hold the pose as long as is comfortable.

5 Come back to standing and repeat the pose on the other side, remembering to alter the cross of the arms.

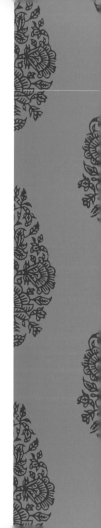

(EAGLE POSE)

Move the arms up, letting the supporting leg straighten slightly. Remain passive as the in-breath enters.

Lengthen and straighten the spine with the exhalation, back of the waist long, pelvis dropping down.

Keep the hips relaxed and almost sit down into them. Drop the weight into the heel of the standing foot.

FOLLOW WITH:

trikonasana
TRIANGLE POSE, PAGES 71–73

parsva konasana
EXTENDED ANGLE, PAGES 74–75

parivrtta trikonasana
TWISTING TRIANGLE, PAGES 98–99

uttanasana
STANDING FORWARD BEND, PAGE 19

malasana (GARLAND POSE)

Combining a forward bend with a squat, this asana works the hips and feet. There are various ways to get into it.

❶ From Tadasana *(see pages 14–15)*: Keep the heels on the ground and extend the arms in front; bend the knees, folding the body forward and down by dropping the pelvis.
From Uttanasana *(see page 19)*: Bend the knees, heels down, and fold in the hips while the trunk stays forward.
From Balasana *(see pages 20–21)*: Take the feet apart, curl the toes under, and, with the hands, push back until the heels reach the ground.

❷ If the heels come up, place a folded blanket under them, and squat again. Keep the knees enough apart for the body to drop between, weight dropping into the heels. The feet splay; without straining the knees, turn them in, balls of the big toes down.

❸ As the trunk lengthens forward, feel a broad stretch across the back of the pelvis. Practice a couple of times, holding as long as is comfortable.

To stay in a squat, the backbone has to lengthen forward. With deep exhalations, the stomach contracting back behind the pubic bone, the length of the spine and therefore the body weight moves forward.

Once forward in the squat, place the arms in Namaste (prayer position), as illustrated; or rest them on the floor in front; or take them back under the knees and rest them on the ground or back of the pelvis.

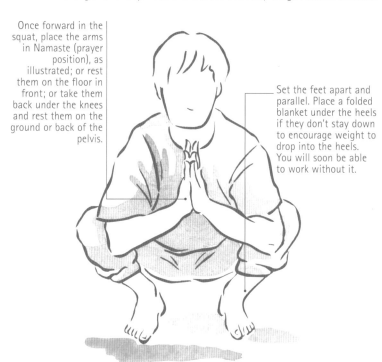

Set the feet apart and parallel. Place a folded blanket under the heels if they don't stay down to encourage weight to drop into the heels. You will soon be able to work without it.

bakasana

(CRANE POSE)

In this hand balance, the arms represent the long legs of the bird, while the top-heavy body hinges in perfect balance above. It is a strong, dynamic pose, gathering energy into the center of the body, with the action of the abdominal muscles massaging the internal organs.

It is not strength that allows you to learn the knack of this pose, but correct technique. Working on Crane Pose can be a lesson in humility: Expect some tumbles, and place a blanket in front of you to protect your head. Stay positive and maintain your sense of humour—you'll experience a wonderful sense of accomplishment when the balance starts to come together.

Cautions: do not try this asana if you have abdominal problems or are pregnant.

FOLLOW WITH:
prasarita padottanasana
STANDING WIDE FORWARD BEND, PAGES 40–41
balasana AND adho mukha svanasana sequence
CHILD POSE AND DOWNWARD FACING DOG, PAGE 20–23

❶ From a squatting position, heels up, place your hands on the ground between the knees, with fingers wide like the foot of a bird. Keep the elbows bent.

❷ Tuck the elbows back and under the knees so that the shins press against the upper arms. Leave the pelvis heavy.

❸ Exhale and, leaving the tail down, let yourself come forward, knees on the back of the arms. Press the knees in to stop them from slipping, and extend the heels backward. Straighten the arms, and round the upper back. Hold as long as is comfortable.

sarvangasana

(SHOULDER STAND—STAGE 1)

This is a preparatory stage for the first inversion in next month's routine: It keeps the neck freer than in the full pose, and allows the spine to lengthen easily. A soothing pose, the balance relaxes the shoulders and begins to open the upper back, so helping muscular or tight shoulders.

You will need a blanket folded to a thickness of 1 inch (2.5cm) and a sturdy chair with a non-slip seat.

Cautions: As with all inverted poses, do not hold if you feel any discomfort, or if pressure builds up behind the face and eyes. See also Cautions, page 158.

❶ Lie at arm's length in front of the chair and place your lower legs on the seat. Place the folded blanket under the head and neck. Hold the chair legs at the bottom.

❷ Exhale and press the heels and feet down on the seat of the chair, letting the pelvis come up.

❸ At first, hold for a short time. Exhale and come down. Rest and repeat.

Once you are used to it, stay in the pose as long as is comfortable. If you desire, stretch up one leg at a time as you exhale. Keep holding the chair legs so that the chair doesn't slip or fall.

Lengthen the spine from the back of the neck to the feet with each exhalation. Push the feet into the chair, taking the pelvis higher.

FOLLOW WITH:
jatara parivartanasana II
SUPINE TWIST II, PAGES 78–79

Keep the arms down by holding the chair legs. Allow the upper back to come in between the shoulderblades and to move with the exhalation, when the chest also widens across the front.

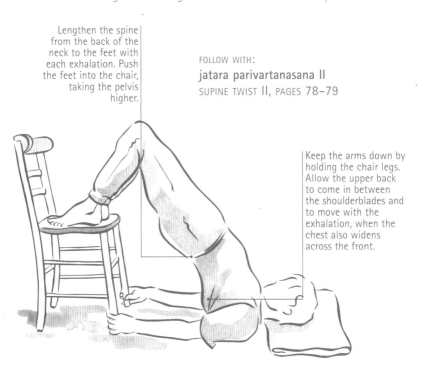

parivrtta upavistha konasana

(TWISTING SEATED ANGLE)

The twist (parivrtta) of Upavistha Konasana *(see pages 82-83)* has a strong lateral stretch that gives a lovely feeling as you open outward, working the hips and enlivening the body. Keep the body weight forward and the sitting bones down, especially the one on the opposite side to the twist.

❶ Sit with legs apart. Exhale and turn the body sideways along the right leg.

❷ Lower the right elbow to the ground inside the right leg and move toward the heel. Bring the left arm up and over, if possible, catching the foot. Exhale, lengthening both sides of the body, and look up toward the top arm.

❸ Breathe in the pose as long as is comfortable, but, to begin with, do not hold for long. Return upright, and repeat the steps on the other side.

Lengthen the side of the body nearest the leg to give a good feeling of traveling along the leg without overstretching the top of the body.

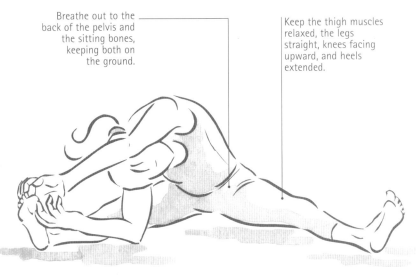

Breathe out to the back of the pelvis and the sitting bones, keeping both on the ground.

Keep the thigh muscles relaxed, the legs straight, knees facing upward, and heels extended.

FOLLOW WITH:
upavistha konasana OPEN ANGLE, PAGES 82–83

pranayama

(SITALI—COOLING BREATH)

Start Pranayama with Ujjayi breathing *(see page 25)*, add in
Kapalabhati *(see pages 123–24)*, return to Ujjayi, then add a
variation *(see pages 86 and 104)*, before finishing with Ujjayi.
This month's new variation is Sitali, the cooling breath.

The technique works by sucking air in across moisture on
the tongue to cool the body and reduce thirst, and was used
by yogis in the desert in ancient times. The method involves
sticking the tongue out, making a round hole with the lips,
and curling up the edges of the tongue into a funnel. If, like
25 percent of us, you can't do this, keep the tongue flat.

❶ Exhale through the nose. At the end, throw
the head back, stretching the front of the throat.
Stick the tongue out and make the funnel.

❷ Inhale through the funnel of the tongue or
over it, making a loud sucking sound. Swallow
the saliva, bringing the head up. Exhale
through the nose gently and easily. Repeat
for several cycles, then return to Ujjayi.

relaxation

Begin in Recuperation Pose I *(see page 26)*, then lengthen the legs out into Savasana *(see page 27)*. Focus on the deep and calming exhalation of the Ujjayi breath *(see page 25)* to ground and relax the back of the body.

❶ Exhale length and inhale broadness. As the inhalation enters, imagine the ribs as a filter through and beyond which the air passes.

❷ Exhale, and as the in-breath enters, feel the front ribs soften, the back ribs expand, and the breath coming up between the shoulders and along the back of the head. Exhale and feel length from the crown of the head to the heels.

❸ After five cycles of conscious breathing, open the eyes, roll to one side, and get up slowly.

the story of yoga

The Mahabharata, consisting of some 100,000 verses, is a rich source of mythology, philosophy, theater, and customs. It was sung, recited, danced, or performed, and in the present day, like the Ramayana, has been filmed and televised to great popular acclaim.

The story is based on a war between two families, the Pandavas and the Kauravas, that was thought to have taken place in 1000 B.C.E., when the Vedic–Aryans were invading northern India.

In the Mahabharata, there is a king who has two sons. The eldest, Dhritarashtra, is blind and so the younger son, Pandu, succeeds to the throne. King Pandu has five sons, the Pandavas, and, when he dies, his blind brother completes their upbringing as noble warriors. Dhritarashtra has 100 sons, the Kauravas, the eldest being the power-hungry Duryodhana. Jealous of his father's affection for the Pandavas, Duryodhana, through trickery, makes Prince Yudhishthira lose both his kingdom and his wife in a game of dice. For this, the five Pandava brothers are banished. At the end of a thirteen-year exile, the virtuous brothers return and demand the restoration of their father's kingdom. When their lawful claim is rejected, the families go to war, and after 18 days of the fiercest battles, the Kauravas are defeated.

Within the story of the Mahabharata is a section called the Bhagavad Gita, or Song of the Lord. It is a spiritually symbolic poem in which

Arjuna, the third of King Pandu's sons, has doubts before going into battle, which he discusses with his charioteer, Krishna. The 8th avatar of the god Vishnu, Krishna reveals to Arjuna not only the higher self or soul of a person (atman), but the method of realizing it through karma yoga, the yoga of action. This positive action, Krishna says in the Bhagavad Gita , is a way to the absolute spirit (brahman) that can be followed by anyone at work in their everyday lives or, in this case, while going into battle. He expounds that it is not action itself that binds humans to the cycle of rebirth, but the selfish intentions behind the actions. If these same actions are performed for the sake of Krishna, who represents the Divine, whoever performs them will be protected.

Krishna also defines three further types of yoga: bhakti yoga, the yoga of love and devotion; jnana yoga, the yoga of knowledge, study, and ascetism; and dhyana yoga, the path of meditation.

The Bhagavad Gita is described as a book of yoga, and its popularity and availability has made it famous in both East and West. By 200 A.D., yoga had been accepted as one of the six systems of Hindu philosophical thought. Before this date, Patanjali codified a system that became known as Raja, or Royal, yoga. It is also called Classical yoga.

month8

Fall is the season to contemplate the concepts of mind and body as you start to work on inverted yoga postures. The main pose for focus in this month's sequence is the shoulder stand Sarvangasana, the mother of all asanas, which enlivens the mind with a fresh flow of blood to the brain while calming and soothing every part of the body: *Sarvanga* is the Sanskrit term for "all the limbs" of the body. Breathing exercises conclude the session with the roaring of the lion breath.

key postures:

warming up (SUPTA PADANGUSTHASANA II)

dhanurasana (BOW POSE)

chaturanga dandasana (PLANK POSE)

vasisthasana (ONE-ARM STAND)

sarvangasana (SHOULDER STAND—STAGES 2 AND 3)

halasana (PLOW POSE)

pranayama (LION BREATH)

relaxation

mind and body

The translation of the Sanskrit word *yoga* is the joining or yoking of mind and body. The definition suggests harmony, the two elements pulling together, like a seesaw finding the point of equilibrium.

Note how some people live in the mind and seem distant from their surroundings. They shrink inward, losing contact even with real objects such as the chair they sit on. Floating through life in this way, without making contact with the physical world, affords only limited choice over actions. Other people are intensely physical—a chair would collapse on them before they noticed its fragility—and they fail to question or see what surrounds them. This, too, is a shrinking away that causes the mind to grow smaller and the silence greater.

Yoga joins the worlds of mind and body. You cannot perform an asana purely with physical strength: The mind traveling inside the body develops the pose. Neither can a pose be performed simply with the mind—there would be no balance nor ground to work from. When mind works with body there is beauty and harmony, and the wisdom of the body refreshes and informs the mind.

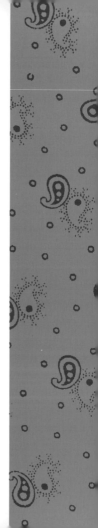

warming up

Start in Recuperation Pose II *(see page 33)* and follow with the supine leg stretches on pages 34–35.

supta padangusthasana II

(LYING DOWN HAND-TO-TOE)

❶ From the single leg stretch *(see above)*, exhale, taking the vertical leg to the side. Keep the opposite hip on the floor so the upper leg releases from the center and away.

❷ Keep the upper leg straight as it moves out, knee facing the shoulder and the arm or belt holding it, heel extended. Turn the thigh inward with the hip to maintain straightness.

❸ With the exhalation, keep both sides of the pelvis heavy. Toward the end of the out-breath, release the leg from the hip out to the side and back toward the hand. On the in-breath, open the back of the knee. Repeat on the other side.

FOLLOW WITH: **supta ardha padmasana** LYING DOWN LOTUS, PAGE 133 **supta gomukhasana** COW LEGS, PAGE 111 AND **supta baddha konasana** ROCKETSHIP POSE, PAGE 91

dhanurasana (BOW POSE)

The bow shape of Dhanurasana is like a seesaw, its fulcrum in the hips and pubic bone. The strings of the bow pull on each end evenly to bend the bow.

Bow Pose is an intense backbend and should follow all of the warming up exercises on the page before.

1 Lie on your stomach, arms by your side, palms up, forehead on the ground. Exhale and practice lengthening the lower back.

2 Bend the lower legs up. Press the hips and groin down, flattening the thighs against the ground. Exhale and reach behind to catch the ankles. Keep the chin in.

3 Exhale, the abdomen contracting back, and evenly lift both ends. Hold briefly. Release on an exhalation and rest before repeating. Use the end of the exhalation to contract the abdomen, protecting the lower back. Release to let the in-breath come easily.

Lengthen the spine with the out-breath, releasing the arms and legs from the trunk without snapping back in the waist.

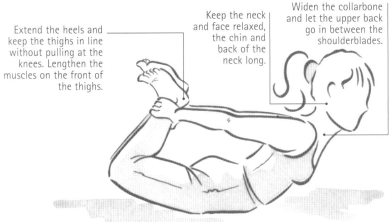

Extend the heels and keep the thighs in line without pulling at the knees. Lengthen the muscles on the front of the thighs.

Keep the neck and face relaxed, the chin and back of the neck long.

Widen the collarbone and let the upper back go in between the shoulderblades.

FOLLOW WITH:

balasana CHILD POSE, PAGES 20-21, eka pada rajakapotasana I ONE LEGGED PIGEON POSE, PAGES 54–55 tadasana MOUNTAIN POSE, PAGES 14–15 FOOT EXERCISE, PAGE 36 namaste 1 REVERSE PRAYER, PAGE 16 virabhadrasana WARRIOR POSE, PAGES 56-57 parivrtta parsvakonasana I TWISTING SIDE ANGLE I, PAGES 118–19 prasarita padottanasana STANDING WIDE FORWARD BEND, PAGES 40–41 balasana AND adho mukha svanasana sequence CHILD POSE AND DOWNWARD FACING DOG, PAGES 20–23

chaturanga dandasana

(PLANK POSE—SEE ILLUSTRATION, PAGE 219)

❶ From Adho Mukha Svanasana (Downward Facing Dog, pages 22–23), step back with both feet and bring the weight forward over the hands as if in a push-up, arms straight, shoulders relaxed, weight in the palms of the hands.

❷ Extend the heels; exhale into the back of the waist to lengthen the spine. Keep the back flat and aligned from back of the skull to heels, chin in, neck long. Come down.

vasisthasana (ONE-ARM STAND)

❶ From Chaturanga Dandasana (Plank Pose, above), roll to the left side, dropping the weight into the left hand. Keep the side of the left foot, with as much of its sole as possible, against the floor.

❷ Place the right leg on top, right foot pressing down on the left foot. Take the right arm off the floor and, exhaling, open the body upward. Develop with the breath as long as is comfortable. Repeat the pose on the other side.

(ONE-ARM STAND)

The exhalation makes the pose straighter, and straightening makes the body lighter.

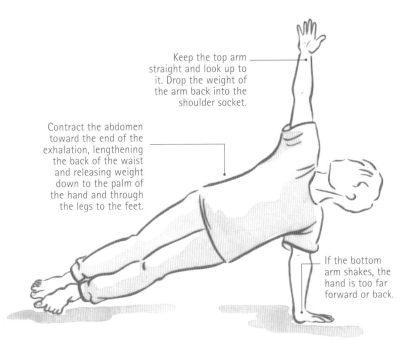

Keep the top arm straight and look up to it. Drop the weight of the arm back into the shoulder socket.

Contract the abdomen toward the end of the exhalation, lengthening the back of the waist and releasing weight down to the palm of the hand and through the legs to the feet.

If the bottom arm shakes, the hand is too far forward or back.

sarvangasana (SHOULDER STAND, STAGE 2)

This calming and soothing pose has a multitude of benefits for many common ailments. It can help the thyroid and parathyroid glands in the neck. In relaxing the legs it helps ease varicose veins, and hip and knee problems. The inversion of the pose strengthens the back, and the reverse of gravity increases the supply of blood to the heart. Since the head remains firm with the chin down, the supply of blood to the brain is regulated, which may cure headaches. The soothing effects of the pose also help relieve nervous conditions and promote a peacefulness that can combat insomnia.

Preparatory work for this pose started with Stage 1 in Month 7 *(see pages 142–43)*. Stages 2 and 3 are illustrated on the following pages. Stage 2 feels quite free on the neck, whereas Stage 3 is more constricted. If at any time in the pose you experience discomfort or a build-up of pressure in the face, neck, or chest, come down. When you go up again, it may have cleared. If not, return to Stage 1 or 2.

Cautions: Seek medical advice before practicing inversions if you suffer from medical problems affecting the head, heart, blood pressure, or eyes. Avoid if you have an arthritic neck or have had metal-support surgery to the spine.

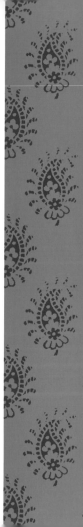

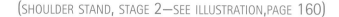

(SHOULDER STAND, STAGE 2—SEE ILLUSTRATION, PAGE 160)

❶ Lie on your back with shoulders and arms on a blanket, palms down. Bend the knees up, keeping the feet flat on the ground. Breathe quietly, aligning the body, feet in front of the hips, shoulders even and relaxed. Keep the chin down and the back of the neck long.

❷ To go up, fold the knees in and, as you exhale, press the arms down. As the abdominals contract, curl the body up.

❸ Bend the elbows and bring your hands under the pelvis.

❹ If the head and neck are uncomfortable, do not move them: Come down, straighten yourself, and go up again. Stay in the pose as long as there is no pressure, but only briefly to begin with.

❺ To come down: Bend the knees, slide the elbows apart, and, still holding the pelvis, unroll. Rest. To correct misalignments, follow with the twist suggested on page 160.

sarvangasana

(SHOULDER STAND, STAGE 2)

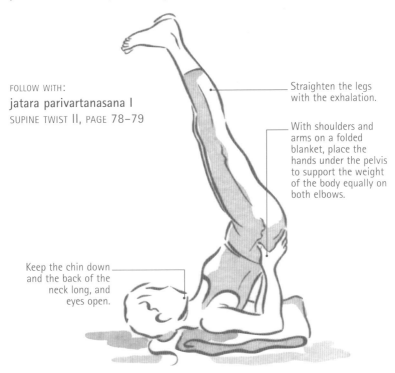

FOLLOW WITH:
jatara parivartanasana I
SUPINE TWIST II, PAGE 78–79

Straighten the legs with the exhalation.

With shoulders and arms on a folded blanket, place the hands under the pelvis to support the weight of the body equally on both elbows.

Keep the chin down and the back of the neck long, and eyes open.

(SHOULDER STAND, STAGE 3—SEE ILLUSTRATION, PAGE 162)

Stage 3 brings the elbows in closer than in Stage 2. The hands move down to the upper back, enabling the torso and legs to become straighter.

1 Follow step 1 in Stage 2 *(see page 159)*, making sure the body is straight before you start to go up. On an out-breath, press down with the arms and curl the body upward.

2 Bend the elbows and bring the palms of the hands flat against the back, little fingers parallel to either side of the spine. Feel the weight distributed across a firm triangle, from shoulders, to elbows, to wrists.

3 As you exhale, lengthen the body up to the feet. Develop with the breath as long as is comfortable.

4 To come down: Place the arms on the floor, palms facing down; bend the knees; and lower the body, unrolling from the top of the spine to the tailbone, the back of the waist touching the floor. Always follow this pose with the twist suggested on page 162.

sarvangasana (SHOULDER STAND, STAGE 3)

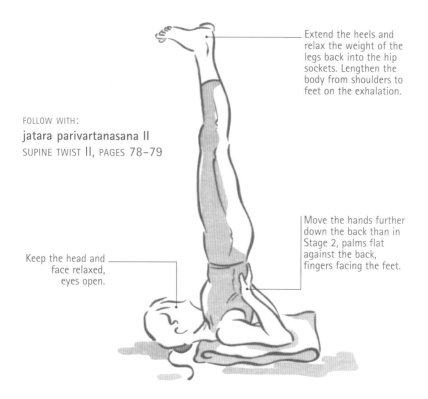

Extend the heels and relax the weight of the legs back into the hip sockets. Lengthen the body from shoulders to feet on the exhalation.

FOLLOW WITH:
jatara parivartanasana II
SUPINE TWIST II, PAGES 78–79

Move the hands further down the back than in Stage 2, palms flat against the back, fingers facing the feet.

Keep the head and face relaxed, eyes open.

halasana (PLOW POSE)

Fall is harvest time, when farmers turn their fields. The earthy plow is celebrated as part of the shoulder balance cycle—*hala* is Sanskrit for "plow"—and like Sarvangasana (Shoulder Stand, pages 158–62), it invokes calm and clarity of thought by relaxing and rejuvenating the brain and the eyes. Start with the preparatory exercise below, and then progress to the full Plow Pose on page 165. See also cautions, page 158, before starting practice.

❶ Place a chair behind your head, at a distance that matches the length of your arms.

❷ Go into Shoulder Stand *(see pages 159–62)*, then exhale and lower the extended legs down to the seat of the chair. Keep the elbows on the ground with the hands against the back. Remain in the pose as long as is comfortable.

❸ To come down: Place the arms on the floor, palms down; bend the knees; and lower the body, unrolling from the top of the spine to the tailbone, back of the waist touching the floor. Follow with the twist suggested on page 164.

halasana (PLOW POSE, STAGE 2)

The Sarvangasana (Shoulder Stand, pages 158–62) and
Halasana (Plow Pose) sequence starts from Plow Pose,
goes into Shoulder Stand and returns to Plow Pose before
unrolling downward.

1 From lying down, let the hips roll up over the head and
rest the feet on a chair *(see page 163)* or the floor. Keep
the shoulders relaxed, the neck long. Bend the arms at the
elbow and place the palms of the hands against the back,
fingers toward the pelvis.

2 Bend the knees and, on an exhalation go into Shoulder
Stand *(see pages 159–162)*.

3 To return to Plow Pose, exhale and lower the extended
legs over your head toward the ground. Exhale and
lengthen the torso from the back of the neck to the
tailbone, hips lifting up. Drop the shoulders back further
to the elbows, allowing the hands to move toward the
upper back. To unroll from Plow Pose: Flatten the arms on
the ground, and unroll, bending the knees toward the end.

(PLOW POSE, STAGE 2)

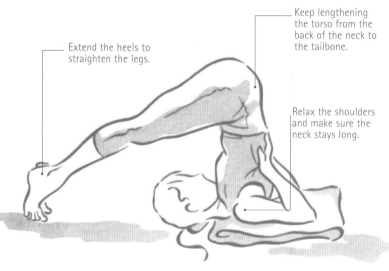

Extend the heels to straighten the legs.

Keep lengthening the torso from the back of the neck to the tailbone.

Relax the shoulders and make sure the neck stays long.

FOLLOW WITH:
jatara parivartanasana II
SUPINE TWIST II, PAGES 78–79

END YOUR ROUTINE WITH:
parivrtta janu sirasana
TWISTING HEAD-TO-KNEE, PAGES 80–81
marichyasana I
SAGE POSE I, PAGES 120-21
pashchimottanasana
SEATED FORWARD BEND, PAGES 44-45

pranayama (LION BREATH)

The roar from the Lion Breath is a powerful and invigorating exhalation; everything goes out from the center.

❶ Sitting cross-legged or in Seated Half Lotus *(see page 122)*, start with Ujjayi breathing *(see page 25)*. Practice Kapalabhati *(see pages 123–24)*, and return to Ujjayi breathing.

❷ For Lion Breath, inhale through the nose until the lungs are full.

❸ Open the mouth wide, stretch the tongue out, roll the eyes up, and stretch out the arms and hands. Exhale with a roar from the back of the throat.

❹ Inhale through the nose gently. Repeat two more times as is comfortable and return to Ujjayi.

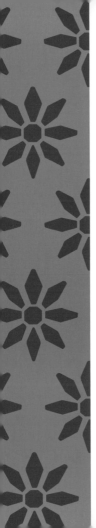

relaxation

Start with Recuperation Pose I *(see page 26)*, then lengthen the legs out into Savasana *(see page 27)*. Having settled the body so that it is relaxed and comfortable, check whether the mind is still busy.

❶ Do not empty the mind or suppress thoughts as this can leave you without options. Feel the stability of the ground beneath you and your body connected to it. Notice thoughts passing through your mind, let them go, and return to the breath, observing it with your mind.

❷ Let the body open back against the ground, the brain relax, and the breath stay easy. Think of the sounds around you as a background, not a distraction. Now be more inside the body, aware of the outer edges around you, and the ground beneath.

❸ After five cycles of conscious breathing, open the eyes, roll to one side, and get up slowly.

the story of yoga

Between 150 B.CE. and 200 A.D., for his dates are not known, the grammarian Patanjali formed the 195 Yoga Sutras. Sutras or threads are concise notes that thread together a series of ideas to make up a system of thought. Patanjali did not originate these ideas, but collected them together from earlier sources. His path of yoga is called Raja, or Classical, yoga, and his work has endured to this day.

The philosophy of Raja yoga is similar to the dualist Samkhya tradition, which teaches that the primordial world was formed from nature or matter (prakrti), which consists of three tendencies (gunas): Lucidity (sattva); energy (rajas); and inertia (tamas). The forming of the world is said to have begun when the balance between the gunas was lost through the appearance of cosmic intelligence (buddhi) that was pure sattva. With further evolution, individual aspects of the real world developed according to the predominance of sattva and tamas, while the remaining gunas, rajas, or energy, was present as the impetus in both, and was also known as prana, the lifeforce.

In human beings, the Samkhya tradition holds that body and mind were made according to the balance of the gunas in unconscious prakrti but the spirit (purusha) was different. Purusha is the conscious eternal self that is similar in quality to the sattvic core of prakrti, but remains a pure and passive onlooker.

Patanjali's path of yoga was formed to realize this self in a state of unification or bliss (samadhi). He formed the Eight Limbs, or steps, of yoga to protect the aspirant yogi from the dangers of misuse, and therefore they start with moral attitudes that are similar to the Ten Commandments in the Christian Bible. The first limb, yama "restraint," controls the contact of the yogi with the outside world and consists of abstinence from harming others, falsehood, theft, incontinence (not being chaste), and greed. Niyama "observances," the second limb, disciplines the yogi's personal behavior and advises purity, contentment, austerity, study, and devotion to the Lord.

The third limb is asana "posture," sitting in a stable position for freeing the mind from disturbances. The fourth limb, pranayama "breath control," regulates the breath: As the flow of breath affects the mind, this promotes the capacity for observation. The fifth limb pratyahara "withdrawal," prepares the mind for spiritual vision by withdrawing its focus the from the senses: External phenomena are considered unimportant since the mind should look inward. In the sixth limb dharanya "concentration," the mind focuses on an internal object of its experience and finds a deeper understanding of it. Dhyana "absorption," the seventh limb, can be reached when concentration becomes spontaneous and the internal object reveals its essence through the supra-consciousness. The eight limb, samadhi, is the illumination and unification of the fully conscious mind with truth.

month9

This month introduces Salamba Sirsasana, the headstand which is sometimes referred to as the king of poses. Just as fall's fruit is ripening, but may not yet be ready to pick, savor the preparatory work for this asana, allowing the pose to ripen and become ready to taste when its flavor is fullest. Other poses continue to extend your growing flexibility with more twists, backbends, and forward bends. Fall is time to explore the concept of fullness and emptying, and this month's breathing exercise rounds off the session by looking at the fullness of the in-breath.

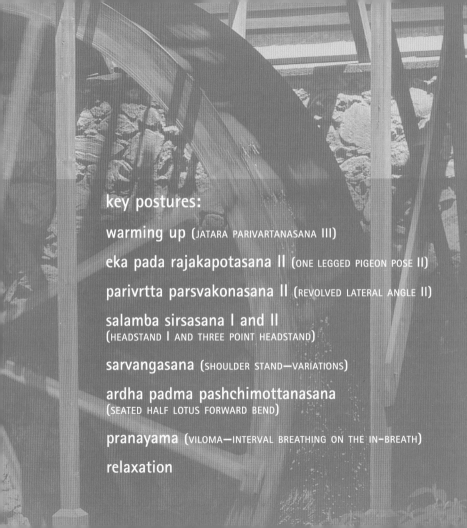

key postures:

warming up (JATARA PARIVARTANASANA III)

eka pada rajakapotasana II (ONE LEGGED PIGEON POSE II)

parivrtta parsvakonasana II (REVOLVED LATERAL ANGLE II)

salamba sirsasana I and II
(HEADSTAND I AND THREE POINT HEADSTAND)

sarvangasana (SHOULDER STAND—VARIATIONS)

ardha padma pashchimottanasana
(SEATED HALF LOTUS FORWARD BEND)

pranayama (VILOMA—INTERVAL BREATHING ON THE IN-BREATH)

relaxation

fullness and emptying

Breathing is a constant cycle of filling and emptying. The same is true of yoga poses. Each time you approach your practice, the pose is there anew, waiting for you. By considering the pose to exist in its own right, rather than being something you "do," you replace an acquisitive attitude with one of involvement, and enter into partnership with the movement, mind and body working together.

Fixing on the pose as an end in itself, and not allowing the pose to teach you and evolve, is as unsatisfactory as devouring an apple without savoring the taste. Use the desire that drove you to grab the apple, or take up yoga, as a motivating force. Harness the strong desire to achieve, to "just do it," to take you forward, but be aware of the dangers of this desire and the frustration it can cause. Yoga works with the evolving body, and it is this progression with understanding that makes it more than a form of physical exercise.

The headstand exists today, and will still be there tomorrow. It is a pose that you pour yourself into, but this is only possible if your base is firm, your hands and elbows down, your neck straight. All of this comes with practice. Therefore, savor the preparatory steps, giving time to the principles that mind and body may not yet have understood. In this way you allow the pose to ripen, and become ready to taste when the flavor is fullest.

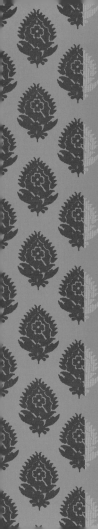

warming up

Start in Recuperation Pose II (page 33) and follow with the supine leg stretches on pages 34–35. Follow with Supta Ardha Padmasana (Lying Down Half Lotus, page 133) and Supta Baddha Konasana (Reclining Bound Angle Pose, page 91), then move on to the asana below.

jatara parivartanasana III
(SUPINE TWIST III)

❶ Lying on your back, fold the knees in, the right hand underneath the thighs. Place the left hand out to the side and look toward it.

❷ Exhale and roll the legs, with the arm still holding them, to the right.

❸ Exhale and lengthen the legs out, the arm still beneath them, heels extending away. Repeat on the other side.

FOLLOW WITH:
balasana CHILD POSE, PAGES 22–2
eka pada rajakapotasana I ONE LEGGED PIGEON POSE I, PAGES 54–55. REPEAT IT A SECOND TIME BEFORE MOVING ON TO THE NEXT STAGE OF THE POSE ON PAGES 174–175.

eka pada rajakapotasana II

(ONE LEGGED PIGEON POSE II)

This is a sideways variation of the full pose with a lovely turning and catching of the back leg. It works the upper back while continuing to warm the hips.

The success of the pose depends on how close to the ground the back of the thigh of the front leg is. If your hip stays high, exhale, come up onto your hands and, breathing out, lengthen the lower back, especially down and under the hip on the bent-leg side. Repeat on the other side and do no more in the pose for now. Continue with Stage I *(see pages 54–55)* until the hip drops more. If the back of your thigh is close to or on the ground, continue as below.

1 Start in Stage I of the pose *(see page 54)*, with the left leg folded under. Exhale and come up onto the hands.

2 Bend the back leg up. Exhale and turn to the right. On another out-breath, catch the back foot with the right hand.

3 Develop the pose with the breath, then repeat on the other side.

[174]

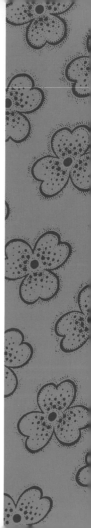

Move the right shoulder blade in and slide the front ribs down and around as you turn into the pose.

Take the left thigh to the ground but do not lean back over it. Keep the weight over the hip of the bent left leg.

FOLLOW WITH:

balasana CHILD POSE, PAGES 20–21

gomukhasana COW POSE, PAGES 114–15

tadasana MOUNTAIN POSE, PAGES 14–15

vrkasana TREE POSE, PAGES 38–39

uttanasana

STANDING FORWARD BEND, PAGE 19

parivrtta parsvakonasana I

REVOLVED LATERAL ANGLE I, PAGES 118–19

Exhale toward the back of the waist, and lengthen the spine downward and upward.

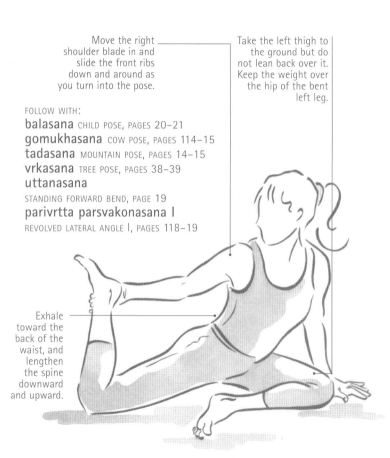

parivrtta parsvakonasana II

(REVOLVED LATERAL ANGLE II)

Like Parivrtta Trikonasana (Twisting Triangle, pages 98–99), this reverse twist turns toward the front leg. The leg seems to block the torso, which needs to lengthen to allow the hand over. Proceed slowly, letting the torso lengthen and turn out. If the bent-leg hip bulks and locks to block the torso, move it down, away· from the shoulder, so there is space for the lumbar spine to turn. The heel under the hip, dispersing weight down, gives stability.

❶ From Ardha Mandalasana (Lunge Pose, pages 100-101), with right knee bent, left leg behind, drop forward over the knee, hands to either side, and relax.

❷ Exhale and turn to the right. Take time to breathe and turn. Place the left hand, on fingertips if necessary, on the ground outside the knee.

❸ Exhale and extend the left heel, straightening the back leg. Exhale, taking the right arm behind the waist or over the head. Come down, and repeat on the other side.

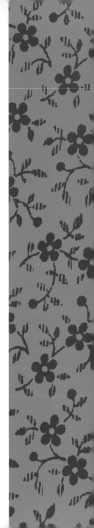

As the right hip and shoulder move away from each other, the torso lies along the line of the thigh as if it had simply turned over.

Exhale toward the back of the waist, and lengthen away from the right hip. Drop this hip down and open the front of the body, taking the shoulder back.

Before placing the left arm outside the bent right knee, use the exhalation to turn the torso more. Stay on fingertips if necessary.

FOLLOW WITH:
balasana CHILD POSE, PAGE 20 AND adho mukha svanasana DOG POSE, PAGE 22.
REPEAT 3 TIMES.

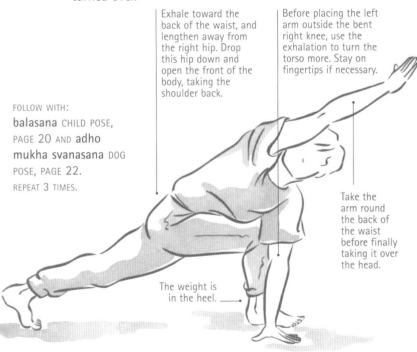

Take the arm round the back of the waist before finally taking it over the head.

The weight is in the heel.

salamba sirsasana

(HEADSTAND)

The Headstand is a challenging, advanced pose, but immensely rewarding. It is easier to learn from a teacher, but if you choose to practice on your own, work carefully, warming up well and keeping your approach calm and quiet. Follow all the preparatory steps opposite, even if you don't attempt the full pose. If you are young and still growing, practice only Salamba Sirsasana II (Three Point Headstand II, pages 182-83).

The benefits of this energizing pose are numerous. It stimulates the pituitary gland and helps boost concentration and confidence while strengthening the arms and wrists. It is useful for the abdominals and varicose veins, and problem hips and knees, too, benefit from being upside down.

Cautions: Seek medical advice before practicing inversions if you suffer from medical or physical problems affecting the head and neck, heart, blood pressure, or eyes, or if you have diabetes. If you are pregnant, do not practice inverted poses unless you were doing so before pregnancy and are stable in them.

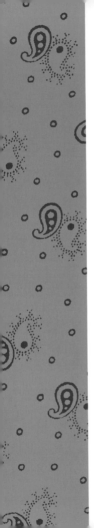

(HEADSTAND, STAGE 1)

❶ Place a mat or blanket down to support the head and arms. Kneel with elbows on the mat, shoulder-width apart.

❷ Clasp the hands, place them on the mat and flatten. Make a triangle with the elbows, the insides strong, wrists flat. This is the firm base.

❸ Feel the weight in the elbows, so heavy they will never come up, and relax the weight of the shoulders down. Flatten the lower arms, wrists turned in and down. Relax the head and neck, and rest the top of the head in front of the hands.

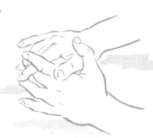

❹ Exhale, straighten the legs, and walk in. Take some weight on the head, but also disperse the weight from elbow to wrist. Check how it feels, then fold down. Relax with arms forward and forehead on the ground. Repeat until the base feels stable.

[179]

salamba sirsasana I

(HEADSTAND, STAGE 2)

The next stage lengthens the upper back to the hips
without bringing the elbows up. Keep the neck straight,
chin in line with the notch in the collarbone. Ensure the
top of the head is not so far back that it pushes on the
neck, nor so far forward that you look at the mat. Keep
the eyes level, looking along the floor. If you feel tension
or pain in the neck or head: You aren't ready to go on.

❶ After following the steps on page 179,
walk in, as before. Exhale, drawing the
abdominal muscles back and lengthening and
straightening the spine to the hips. Bring the
hips over the head, keeping the elbows firm.

❷ Exhale, bend the knees, and, as the elbows
go down, lift the feet off the ground. Be sure
to lift rather than push.

❸ Stay as illustrated. Come down,
and kneel forward with arms loose.

(HEADSTAND, STAGE 3)

❶ After following the steps on page 180, walk into the pose again. Exhale and lengthen, bringing the hips over the head with the elbows down and the triangle stable. Bend the knees slightly, and on another exhalation, lift the legs and lengthen them above you.

❷ Exhale and lengthen up to the heels. Think about the heavy triangle of elbows and wrists, and the exhalation aligning you.

❸ To come down: Bend the knees and descend slowly. Rest, kneeling forward, arms in front, to relax the neck. To finish, release the neck with one of the poses suggested.

FOLLOW WITH:
sarvangasana SHOULDER STAND STAGE 1, PAGES 142–43 STAGES 2 OR 3, PAGES 158–62 VARIATIONS OR adho mukha svanasana DOWNWARD FACING DOG, PAGES 22-23

salamba sirsasana II

(THREE POINT HEADSTAND)

Many people find this variation of the Headstand easier.
Start by placing a folded blanket over a non-slip mat.

1 From kneeling, place the hands, shoulder-width apart,
on the non-slip mat under the edge of the blanket. Spread
the fingers, palms wide and flat against the ground. Leave
the elbows down, relax the shoulders, and become quiet.

2 Bring the elbows up and place your head on the blanket
to form the apex of a triangle with the hands. Exhale and
draw the elbows in over the hands, wrists straight.

3 On an out-breath, straighten the legs and walk in until
the hips are above the head without the palms coming up.

4 Exhale and take the legs up. Keep the elbows in over
the wrists. Exhale and lengthen to the feet.

5 To come down: Bend the knees and descend slowly,
with control. Kneel forward with arms in front, and rest.

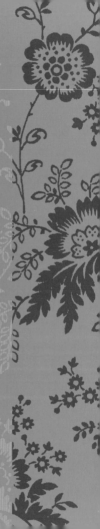

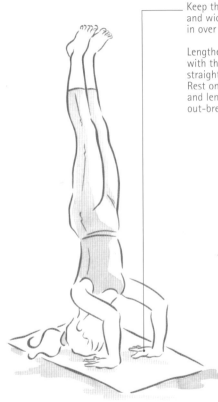

Keep the hands flat
and wide, the elbows
in over the wrists.

Lengthen to the feet
with the out-breath to
straighten the pose.
Rest on the in-breath
and lengthen on the
out-breath.

TO CORRECT MISALIGNMENT,
ALWAYS FOLLOW HEADSTAND WITH:
sarvangasana SHOULDER
STAND STAGES 2 OR 3, PAGES
158–62 OR adho mukha
svanasana DOWNWARD
FACING DOG, PAGES 22–23

sarvangasana

(SHOULDER STAND—VARIATIONS)

In this approach to the Shoulder Stand *(see pages 158–62)*, start in Plow Pose (Halasana, pages 163–65) before bending the knees and going up into the shoulder balance. Once in the pose, try one or all of the leg variations opposite.

If Sarvangasana is a regular part of your yoga practice, you may benefit from using a belt placed above the elbows to keep the elbows in and make lengthening upward easier. Make the belt slightly wider than the shoulders and not too tight, then put it on while in Plow Pose. Go up into the shoulder balance, and when you have finished, drop your legs back into Plow Pose and remove the belt before unrolling down.

After practicing the variations, come down into Plow Pose, place the arms on the ground and unroll, bending the knees toward the end.

(SHOULDER STAND—VARIATIONS)

❶ In Shoulder Stand *(see pages 159–62)*, exhale and release one leg down while keeping the other vertical and steady. The downward leg remains straight, as does the pelvis, so although the leg won't touch the ground, it is fully relaxed in the hip. Hold for several cycles of breath, then bring the leg back up, moving on an out-breath.

❷ In Shoulder Stand *(see pages 159–62)*, exhale and take the legs apart. Hold for several cycles of breath, then bring the legs back together, moving on an out-breath.

❸ In Shoulder Stand *(see pages 159–62)*, exhale and place the soles of the feet together in Baddha Konasana (Cobbler's Pose, pages 102-103). Hold for several cycles of breath, then extend the legs again on an out-breath.

FOLLOW WITH:
halasana PLOW POSE, PAGES 163–65
jatara parivartanasana II
SUPINE TWIST II, PAGE 78–79

ardha padma pashchimottanasana

(SEATED HALF LOTUS FORWARD BEND)

Lengthen forward in Baddha Konasana (Cobbler's Pose, pages 102–103) before going into this pose. Here, having the foot in Half Lotus eases the forward bend since it holds the thigh of the long leg down and releases the forward tilt of the pelvis. If you have difficulty getting the leg into Half Lotus, don't despair; instead repeat Janu Shirshasana (Seated Head-to-Knee, pages 80–81).

❶ Sit with the right leg straight in front. Take the left foot, left hand under the ankle, right hand behind the toes, and draw the foot up the left thigh as near to the groin as able.

❷ Place the hands on the ground behind for support, and relax the hips and legs. Exhale and extend upright.

❸ Exhale, feeling the sitting bones, and lengthen upward. Keep the weight equal over the hip of the half-lotus side, exhale, and lengthen forward. Repeat on the other side.

The lotus leg comes from an outward rotation of the hip and there is no strain in the knee. In the pose, receive the in-breath passively and lengthen on the out-breath.

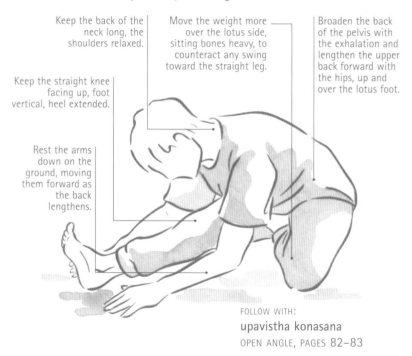

Keep the back of the neck long, the shoulders relaxed.

Move the weight more over the lotus side, sitting bones heavy, to counteract any swing toward the straight leg.

Broaden the back of the pelvis with the exhalation and lengthen the upper back forward with the hips, up and over the lotus foot.

Keep the straight knee facing up, foot vertical, heel extended.

Rest the arms down on the ground, moving them forward as the back lengthens.

FOLLOW WITH:
upavistha konasana
OPEN ANGLE, PAGES 82–83

pranayama

(VILOMA—INTERVAL BREATHING ON THE IN-BREATH)

Pausing on the in-breath gives an increasing fullness that expands inside the body while the shoulders stay relaxed and quiet. It is vital to feel grounded, weight sinking down.

❶ Start with Ujjayi breathing *(see page 25)*, move on to Kapalabhati *(see pages 123–24)*, then return to Ujjayi.

❷ Let the inhalation enter; exhale. At the end of the out-breath, let a little in-breath enter, and pause, feeling quiet.

❸ Let in the rest of the in-breath, and exhale. Repeat the single pause on the in-breath for five inhalations, as comfortable, exhaling between. End the session with Ujjayi.

❹ Next day, increase the pauses to two. At the end of the exhalation, let in a little in-breath and pause; let in a little more and pause; let in the remaining in-breath and exhale. Increase the length of the pause to the count of three with a count of two between. Do not pause at the top of the exhalation. When able, increase to three pauses.

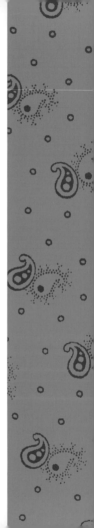

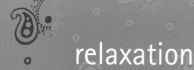

relaxation

Start in Recuperation Pose I *(see page 26)* and when you feel ready, lengthen the legs into Savasana *(see page 27)*. The body is relaxed and the fullness of the in-breath has left you feeling lighter and more open. Exhale deeply, contracting the abdomen back toward the spine like a bowl that has been scraped clean. Feel the back of the body heavier and let the front ribs grow lighter, the in-breath traveling further behind, expanding the sides and back of the body. Let the mind relax and the breath become easy.

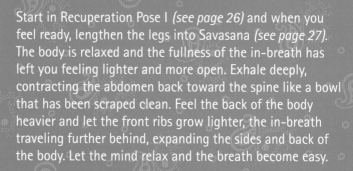

❶ Smooth out the face, opening the forehead and keeping the space between the eyebrows wide.

❷ As the in-breath comes, imagine it as a pail of water filling slowly to the brim.

❸ As you exhale, feel the ground supporting every part of your body, nurturing you as you relax.

❹ After five cycles of conscious breathing, open the eyes, roll to one side, and get up slowly.

the story of yoga

From the 2nd century B.C.E. to the third century A.D., India was ruled by a succession of invaders and dynasties, and it was only with Chandragupta in 320 A.D. that India's political life settled, and a flowering of art, architecture, literature, and philosophy came about.

During the Gupta era, and before the invasion of the Islamic Moguls, the old Brahmanical religion developed into Hinduism. A system of philosophy emerged that was more influential than the Samkhya dualist approach: The non-dualism of Advaita Vedanta. This way of thinking developed from the Upanishad texts with a concept of brahman as the supreme reality.

The philosopher Shankara (c.788–820 A.D.) was born in western Malabar, south India. He studied yoga with other gurus and wrote many works on non-dualism. These expounded the non-theistic view that everything in the world, material, mental, and spiritual, contains the essence of brahman—pure existence and pure consciousness—and that the spirit or soul of human beings, known as atman, is essentially the same as brahman. Shankara taught that what humans experience as themselves is not the pure self of atman, but the illusory experience of separateness (jivatman). The pure spirit of atman is surrounded by layers, one the body, another the mind, and other various forms of conscious-ness. By penetrating these layers with meditation, the philosopher wrote, the kernel of the identical atman and brahman could be revealed. The concept of layers covering the essential spirit of the body was also present in Tantric literature, which held that five layers of increasingly fine particles of energy surround the kernel of spirituality.

Hindu Tantrism emerged during the period of the 6th to 14th centuries A.D. as a yoga of action. It looked for a way to integrate ordinary life within the loftier ideals of Advaita Vedanta, so that it would not be necessary to give up all pleasures in order to become enlightened. Tantrism accepted the non-dualist view that the real world had the same essence as the transcendental reality, but, in the Tantric philosophy, enlightenment did not have to transcend reality; it could co-exist and be improved by it.

Within Tantrism, yoga exercises were used as a direct method of gaining spiritual experience alongside the use of sound (mantra), sight (yantra or mandala), light (trataka), and sexual energy. The latter has given Tantrism a dubious reputation, but it was just one aspect of a literature that, like Ayurvedic medicine, examined the interactive nature of mind and body to find health and well-being. This in turn influenced Hatha yoga.

section III index

winter

fruition

Fall's abundance, the rich harvests of the year, the leaves turning through their myriad of colours reflect the variety of yoga poses you have learned. In October, November and December, more new poses provide different ways of turning and stretching. Again these routines are interspersed with poses you have already done to make a full complement of exercise for each month. As you get to know the new poses you will have all that you need for beginning to form your own way of practice, and to take this year into the next.

month 10

month 11

month 12

month 10

At the start of a new season, the topic for thought is the wave of the breath, that, like yoga itself, balances work and rest to conserve precious energy—something that is particularly important in the cold winter months. The main asana for the month, the full backarch, Wheel Pose, is performed with the wave of the breath, which combines with firm grounding to enable the body to arch up easily. The pose is counter-balanced by Tortoise Pose, a forward bend, and the graceful balance, Half Moon Pose. Pranayama work introduces a new element to breathing—sound—with the vibrational breath, Bhramari.

key postures:

warming up (BHAIRAVASANA)

ardha chandrasana (HALF MOON POSE)

parivrtta ardha chandrasana (REVOLVED HALF MOON)

urdhva dhanurasana (WHEEL POSE)

kurmasana (TORTOISE POSE)

pranayama (BHRAMARI—BEE BREATH)

relaxation

the wave of the breath

Yoga advises rest between the poses and the counterbalance of one pose with another. Stimulating backarches, for example, are always followed by soothing forward bends. Within the breath itself exists a similar pattern of rest and work, and it is through resting on the in-breath that energy is maintained. In this way, yoga practice should not tire you; rather, it energizes mind and body.

A wave gathers energy in constant motion, coming and going across the ocean before spending itself on the beach. Then the wave withdraws, resting, before the next one arrives in a continuous and maintained movement. In breathing, the exhalation is like the wave, while the inhalation resembles the undertow, the re-gathering of energy.

Performing the poses with the exhalation (that releases the spine, making movement easier) is like being a surfer, catching the moment of the wave at a curve of energy when movement is fluid. Think about catching this wave of energy offered by the out-breath especially when performing the Wheel Pose *(see pages 202-205)*, in which the backarch harnesses the curve of energy to release and lengthen the spine while simultaneously being connected by gravity to the stability of the ground. After this burst of energy comes the regenerative in-breath, and so the rhythm of the body continues.

warming up

Start in Recuperation Pose II (page 33) and follow with the supine leg stretches on pages 34–35, then the pose below. It is not a pose to push: Allow breath and gravity to take their course.

bhairavasana (HALF YOGA SLEEPING POSE)

❶ Lie on your back in Recuperation Pose II *(see page 33)*. Bend in the right leg, letting the knee drop to the side. Put the right arm inside the right knee and around the back of the lower leg.

❷ Let the knee drop back toward the shoulder, the thigh close to the side of the body. Keep the knee and lower leg relaxed so that you could move it up and down if desired. Exhale to lengthen the lower back, while the bent leg drops back, left side of the pelvis coming up slightly.

FOLLOW WITH:
supta arha pamasana LYING DOWN HALF LOTUS, PAGE 133 ON THE LEFT SIDE AND THEN REPEAT THE SEQUENCE FROM STEP 1 ON THE RIGHT SIDE.

FOLLOW WITH:

vajrasana THUNDERBOLT POSE, PAGE 52
parivrtta vajrasana THUNDERBOLT TWIST, PAGE 53
tadasana MOUNTAIN POSE, PAGES 14-15
virabhadrasana WARRIOR POSE, PAGES 56-57
uttanasana STANDING FORWARD BEND, PAGE 19

ardha chandrasana

(HALF MOON POSE)

This graceful pose gives a wonderfully freeing feeling as the body opens out in all directions. Before starting, check that your hands touch the ground in Uttanasana (Standing Forward Bend, page 19). If they don't, practice with your lower hand resting on an upturned bucket or prop of similar height. Set it slightly outside the leg you balance on.

If you find the balance difficult, try working against a wall. Stand with the left hip against the wall and bend forward, hands to the ground in front. Take the right leg up, opening and turning back against the wall, and extending the right arm. Turn around and repeat on the other side.

ardha chandrasana

(HALF MOON POSE—SEE ILLUSTRATION, PAGE 200)

1 From Tadasana *(see pages 14-15)*, exhale and bend forward. Place the fingertips of both hands lightly on the floor, a little way in front of you and slightly wider than your feet. Keep the weight in the heels, the legs straight.

2 Exhale and extend the right leg behind. Breathe to establish the line of the leg (aligned with the body), weight in the supporting left heel.

3 Exhale and turn the body to the right. As the right arm comes off the ground, align it with the line of the body.

4 Exhale and take the arm up. Turn the head to look up toward the hand.

5 Hold as long as possible, breathing out to all the body's extremities—the hands, feet, and the crown of the head— as if forming the shape of a star. Come down and repeat on the other side.

ardha chandrasana

(HALF MOON POSE)

FOLLOW WITH:
malasana GARLAND POSE, PAGES 138-39
bakasana CRANE POSE, PAGES 140-41
balasana AND adho mukha
svanasana CHILD POSE AND DOWNWARD FACING DOG,
PAGE 20-23

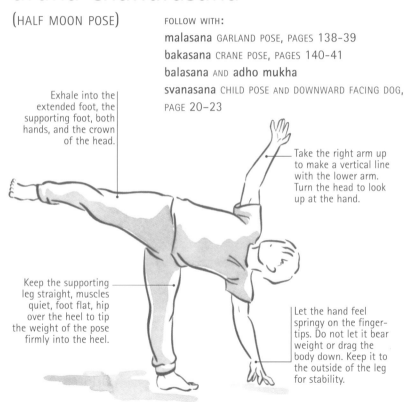

Exhale into the extended foot, the supporting foot, both hands, and the crown of the head.

Take the right arm up to make a vertical line with the lower arm. Turn the head to look up at the hand.

Keep the supporting leg straight, muscles quiet, foot flat, hip over the heel to tip the weight of the pose firmly into the heel.

Let the hand feel springy on the fingertips. Do not let it bear weight or drag the body down. Keep it to the outside of the leg for stability.

parivrtta ardha chandrasana (REVOLVED HALF MOON)

Before continuing with the follow-on poses, reverse the previous pose into a twist. It gives a more intense turn, but can be easier to hold, since the balance is between opposite limbs, and the hip moves over the supporting leg. Because this hip takes the pressure as it turns, the back leg and body need to lift, becoming lighter and longer with the exhalation. If you find the balance tricky, work against a wall, or rest the lower hand, as explained on page 198.

1 From Tadasana *(see pages 14-15)*, bend forward and place the fingertips down in front. Exhale and take the right leg back.

2 Exhale; turn the body toward the left leg, leaving the right hand down. Take the left arm up and look toward it.

3 Exhale to the outer points of the body—the arms, legs, and head. Come down and repeat on the other side.

urdhva dhanurasana (WHEEL POSE)

Invigorating and rejuvenating, Wheel Pose is a wonderful expression of flexibility working in tandem with the breath. It is an advanced pose, and if it takes time to achieve the feeling of energy, practice the previous backarches: Setu Bandha Sarvangasana (Bridge Pose Half Backarch, pages 76–77), or Ushtrasana (Camel Pose, pages 134–35). Make sure the body has been well warmed by this month's previous poses before starting Wheel Pose.

Cautions: seek medical advice before practicing if you have back or disk problems, a hernia, detached retina, or epilepsy.

(WHEEL POSE, STAGE 1)

❶ Lie flat, knees bent up. Take the arms over the head and place the hands behind the shoulders.

❷ Breathe, grounding the body and feeling the wave of the breath as you exhale. Feel the feet and hands as the roots of the pose, from which, with the breath, the body releases up.

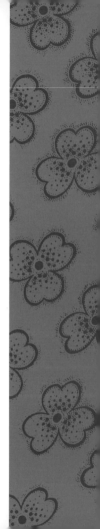

(WHEEL POSE, STAGE 1)

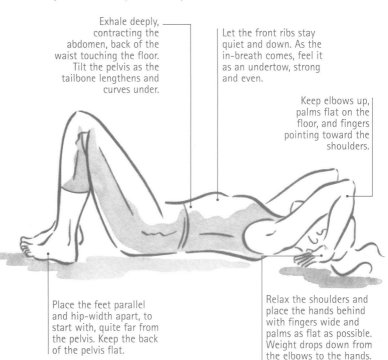

Exhale deeply, contracting the abdomen, back of the waist touching the floor. Tilt the pelvis as the tailbone lengthens and curves under.

Let the front ribs stay quiet and down. As the in-breath comes, feel it as an undertow, strong and even.

Keep elbows up, palms flat on the floor, and fingers pointing toward the shoulders.

Place the feet parallel and hip-width apart, to start with, quite far from the pelvis. Keep the back of the pelvis flat.

Relax the shoulders and place the hands behind with fingers wide and palms as flat as possible. Weight drops down from the elbows to the hands. Keep both hands and feet quiet against the ground.

urdhva dhanurasana

(WHEEL POSE, STAGE 2)

This pose is easier to do on a non-slip mat.

❶ From Stage 1 *(see pages 204-205)* as the weight drops downward, let an in-breath enter fully.

❷ Exhale and, as the back of the waist touches the ground, scoop the pelvis up. Drop the weight into the feet and hands, and let the body come up. Work to keep both sides of the body equal. If the knees splay outward, loosely tie a belt above the knees at hip-width. If the palms of the hands stay high, place a folded mat beneath the wrists.

❸ Hold the pose for one cycle of breath, more if possible. Come down on the out-breath. Fold the knees into the chest. Rest, then repeat. Work up to a maximum of five repetitions, resting with knees folded in after each one.

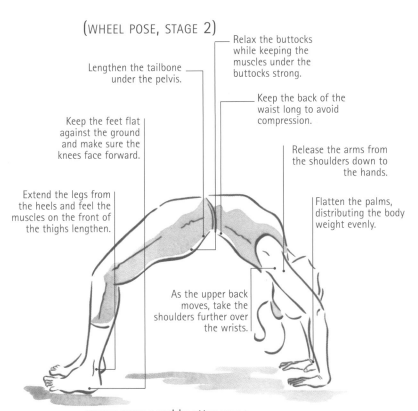

(WHEEL POSE, STAGE 2)

Relax the buttocks while keeping the muscles under the buttocks strong.

Lengthen the tailbone under the pelvis.

Keep the back of the waist long to avoid compression.

Keep the feet flat against the ground and make sure the knees face forward.

Release the arms from the shoulders down to the hands.

Extend the legs from the heels and feel the muscles on the front of the thighs lengthen.

Flatten the palms, distributing the body weight evenly.

As the upper back moves, take the shoulders further over the wrists.

FOLLOW WITH: **paschimottanasana**
SITTING FORWARD BEND, PAGES 42–43 OR **kurmasana** PAGE 206

[205]

kurmasana (TORTOISE POSE)

You need a strong forward bend after a backarch, and
Tortoise is the most intense of these. Go into the pose
slowly and only as far as flexibility allows.

❶ Sit with knees bent, feet hip-width apart in front.

❷ Exhale, leaving the hips and sitting bones heavy, and
lengthen up and forward, coming closer to the thighs and
dropping the elbows between the knees. If you go no further,
this lengthens the back and is restful after a backarch.

❸ Continue lengthening forward. When the knees are above
the shoulders, turn the arms to reach out sideways under
the knees, palms down. Let the feet go forward, but keep
the knees close to the trunk. Exhaling, flatten down further.

❹ (Not illustrated.) Take the arms behind, palms upward,
then catching each other, feet crossing at the ankles, head
on the floor. Vary the cross of the ankles.

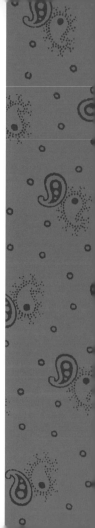

Take this pose slowly, never pushing further than your level of flexibility allows.

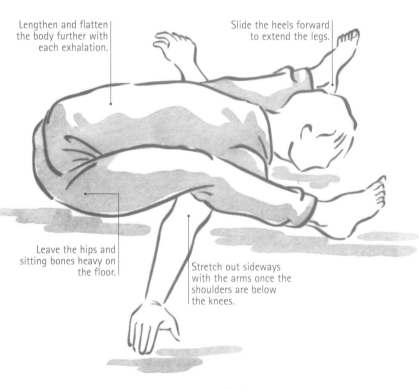

Lengthen and flatten the body further with each exhalation.

Slide the heels forward to extend the legs.

Leave the hips and sitting bones heavy on the floor.

Stretch out sideways with the arms once the shoulders are below the knees.

pranayama

(BHRAMARI—BEE BREATH)

This vibration breath is like the buzzing of a bee. It warms the body, relaxes and energizes, and massages the spine from the inside. The vibrations also help align the spine, (feel the full effect by sitting straight). It's common to burst out laughing when you start learning to buzz!

The vibration breath is performed on the exhalation. First feel the buzz on the front of the lips. Then take it further inside to the back of the head and down the inside of the throat. Finally, feel the vibration traveling down the spine.

1 Sitting straight, start with Ujjayi breathing *(see page 25)*, move on to Kapalabhati *(see pages 123–24)*, then return to the Ujjayi breath.

2 Let an in-breath enter quietly. Exhale, buzzing slowly, the lips vibrating. Focus on the vibration, not the sound.

3 Let in another in-breath and, on the next exhalation, buzz. Continue buzzing on each exhalation for several cycles before returning to Ujjayi breathing.

relaxation

Start in Recuperation Pose I *(see page 26)*, then lengthen
into Savasana *(see page 27)*. The buzzing inside the body
has made you more open: Take a moment to enjoy the
space within and the movement of breath. Feel the back of
the body against the floor, the back of the waist
lengthening with the exhalation, the hips wide, the back of
the legs heavy. Relax the shoulders; calm the head and face.

1 Exhale a little deeper, feeling the breath drop behind
the stomach and almost disappear. Let the in-breath enter
that space and move back up the body.

2 Feel the abundance of space in the body, the front ribs
softening, the exhalation dropping further to the spine.

3 Exhale to the edges of the body, letting the breath undo
tension in the deepest corners. As it comes, allow the in-
breath to fill the spaces and open them further.

4 After five cycles of conscious breathing, open the eyes,
roll to one side, and get up slowly.

the story of yoga

Ramanuja (1017–1137 A.D.) disagreed with Shankara's Advaita Vedantic view of the impersonal nature of brahman, the supreme reality, and replaced it with a notion of the Divine. In this new way of thinking, the liberated person attained a constant co-relationship with the Divine that was a continuous devotion of love. The purpose of meditation in this system was to generate such love, and devotion (bhakti) yoga was the form of meditation Ramanuja prescribed, making Advaita Vedanta more vibrant and devotional.

Arab traders—Muslims from the Turkish peoples—had been raiding India from the West since the 7th century A.D., and in the 11th century a new group of invaders settled in the Punjab in northwest India. By the 12th century, Turkish Sultanates had been established in Delhi, and as the new rulers did not demand conversion to Islam of the Indian population, a fruitful interchange of cultures ensued.

Sufism, a mystical movement within Islam seeking unity with God through fervent worship, took on board the devotionalism of Ramanuja's Bhakti yoga, and Kabir, a Muslim weaver, integrated the Sufi with the Bhakti traditions, influencing Guru Nanak (1469–1538), who founded the Sikh religion. Nanak believed in one transcendent divinity, the name of which could be brahman or Allah, and taught that the true essence of god could be revealed through meditation on any of the names for God.

Growing out of the Tantric yoga of action, the tradition of Hatha yoga began in the 10th century, and was written down in the Hatha Yoga Pradipika (Torch of Hatha Yoga) in the mid-14th century by yoga master, Svatmarama. The Pradipika was a practical guide to the philosophy and techniques that integrated body and mind for the purpose of understanding the spiritual inner self. Svatmarama also wished to realize the Raja yoga of Patanjali.

The Pradipika describes asanas and pranayama in much greater depth than Patanjali's Yoga Sutras, and practical exercises were also developed to affect the subtle body—by this time, Tantric, Hatha, and Kundalini yoga all had an established physiology of the inner body. Within the subtle body, they taught, exists a system of currents (nadis) and seven chakras—centers of energy—that bear similarities to the nervous and endocrine systems of orthodox western medicine. The purpose of yoga was to awaken, through pranayama, the psychic force of kundalini (the sleeping serpent) at the base of the spine, and force its energy through the chakras up the central channel of the sushumna that lies along the spine.

Kundalini, the female principle, on reaching the top chakra at the crown of the head, became united with the male principle of the god Shiva, bringing about a transformation of consciousness.

month 11

During winter, the days are shorter, so celebrate dawn and the precious light it brings with the Sun Salutation, a series of movements that exercises the entire body. Combined with shoulder balance and a twist, it contains all the movements the spine needs to maintain health and well-being. Breathing examines Khumbhaka, the retention breath, which offers a unique moment of concentrated stillness and clarity.

key postures:

warming up

surya namaskar (SUN SALUTATION)

marichyasana II (SAGE TWIST II)

pranayama (KHUMBHAKA—RETENTION BREATH)

relaxation

sequence, flow, and body image

The end of the year brings with it a thoughtful quality that is not unpleasant. Work has been done, the wood cut and stacked, or the central heating system overhauled. Or perhaps neither. Perhaps you are still rushing to catch up, to mend the leak in the roof, or fix the window that won't shut. This is also part of the cycle, and however much you may wish you were someone who tackled these types of things, celebrate the fact that you're not. The beauty of individuals is in variety, and for each of us, different gifts and problems offer a way toward self-development.

You come to yoga as you are, and without any special attributes. Yoga offers no judgments, only a flow, a current of consecutive actions, and your own personal current may be elusive and difficult to find. You cannot buy it, nor force it, nor pretend it's there.

Yoga encourages introspection by working on the body from the inside out. It allows you to become friends with your body and learn to love yourself. This is not a selfish self that denies all others, or any particular self—it is simply a self, varied in its quirks and mannerisms, and infinitely interesting. And all encased in the ultimate packaging: Simple skin and bone.

warming up

The Sun Salutation sequence of poses on pages 216–22 is a warming-up exercise in itself, but it can also help to warm the body before your practice.

The following is an overview of the warm-up options to select from:

surya namaskar

(SUN SALUTATION)

This sequence of 12 postures is traditionally performed 12 times, alternating on each side of the body, in the morning, as the name suggests. The sequence of poses is coordinated with the cycle of breath, and the movements performed with the inhalation are as relaxed and grounded as those done on the exhalation.

You have seen all the poses before except Eight Point Pose *(see page 219)*, but revise each one briefly before you start, especially poses 5 and 6. To begin with, perform each movement on the exhalation, keeping your breathing smooth, natural, and without strain. When familiar with the routine, you will find your movements flowing easily with the length and rhythm of both in- and out-breaths.

Think of the sequences in pairs, practicing the first one with the right leg stepping back and the next one with the left. Keep rooted in the feet, back of the waist long.

To start with an easier variation, substitute poses 6 and 7 with Balasana (Child Pose, pages 20–21). Then come up to hands and knees, inhale, and curl the toes under. Rejoin the sequence by exhaling into pose 8.

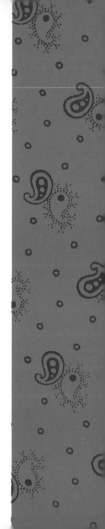

(SUN SALUTATION)

Starting with the right leg:

❶ tadasana
(MOUNTAIN POSE, PAGES 14-15)
—arms in namaste

Stand in Tadasana, hands in Namaste (prayer), lower arms down, palms together, away from the body. Exhale; drop the hands and arms to the sides.

❷ tadasana—arms up

Inhale, and take the arms above the head. Leave the shoulders down and feel the weight of the body in the heels.

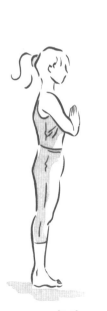

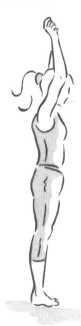

❸ uttanasana
(STANDING FORWARD BEND, PAGE 19)
Exhale, bending forward, knees
straight.

❹ ardha mandalasana
(LUNGE POSE, PAGES 100–101)
Inhale, bend the knees and
step back with the right leg.
Keep the left heel down.

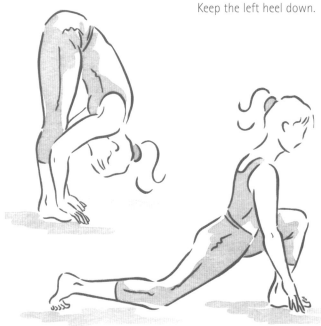

❺ chaturanga dandasana (PLANK POSE, PAGE 156)
Pause at the top of the inhalation, taking the left
leg back to join the right leg, straightening the
legs, extending the heels, and bringing the weight
over the wrists.

❻ astanga namaskar (EIGHT POINT POSE)
Exhale, bend the knees down, bend the elbows, and drop the chest
and chin to the ground so that you have eight points on the floor:
2 feet, 2 knees, 1 chest, 1 chin, and 2 hands.

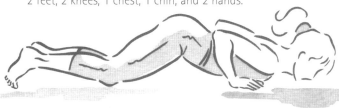

❼ bhujangasana
(COBRA POSE, PAGES 112–13)
Flatten the tail down, pelvis on the ground,
slide between the hands, and inhale up into
Cobra Pose.

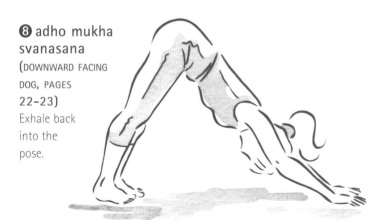

❽ adho mukha svanasana
(DOWNWARD FACING
DOG, PAGES
22–23)
Exhale back
into the
pose.

❾ ardha mandalasana
(LUNGE POSE, PAGES 100–101)
Inhale and bring the right leg
forward, keeping the heel down.

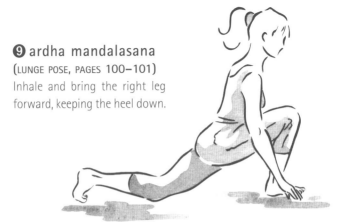

❿ uttanasana
(STANDING FORWARD BEND, PAGE 19)
Exhale and bring the left leg up to
join the right in the
forward bend, knees straight.

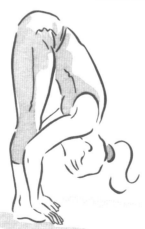

⑪ tadasana
(MOUNTAIN POSE, PAGES 14–15)
—arms up
Inhale; take the hands, backs together, up through the center to above the head, then apart.

⑫ tadasana—hands in namaste
Exhale, taking each arm out to the side and describing the two sides of a circle before coming back to the center in Namaste.

Repeat the sequence, starting with the left leg.

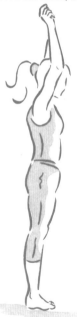

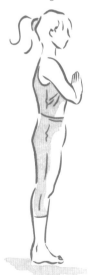

mini routine

If short of time, follow the Sun Salutation with pranayama, relaxation, or continue with the following:

tadasana MOUNTAIN POSE, PAGES 14–15 WITH COW ARMS, PAGE 70
parivrtta parsvakonasana I AND **II** TWISTING SIDE ANGLES I AND II, PAGES 118–19 AND 176–77
prasarita padottanasana STANDING WIDE FORWARD BEND, PAGES 42–43
salamba sirsasana I AND **II** HEAD STANDS I AND II, PAGES 178–83
sarvangasana SHOULDER STAND, PAGES 158–62 AND **halasana** PLOW POSE, PAGES 163–65 INCLUDING VARIATIONS PAGES 184–85
jatara parivartanasana II SUPINE TWIST II, PAGES 78–79
setu bandha sarvangasana BRIDGE POSE, PAGES 76–77
urdva dhanurasana WHEEL POSE, PAGES 202–205
parivrtta janu shirshasana TWISTING HEAD-TO-KNEE, PAGES 58–59
marichyasana I AND **II** SAGE POSE I AND II, PAGES 120–21 AND 224–225
upavistha konasana OPEN ANGLE, PAGES 82–83

marichyasana II

(SAGE TWIST II)

This advanced pose is much more intense than the first Sage Pose *(see pages 120-21)*. Turning to the outside of the bent knee and wrapping the arms around creates a compact contortion of the body in which the abdominal muscles and internal organs also turn. To practice the pose in a more open way, turn to the outside of the knee, take the back arm behind, and extend the front arm forward outside the bent knee; look over the back shoulder.

❶ Sit with the left leg straight and the right knee bent.

❷ Breathe out and turn to the right, stretching the left arm out. Breathe, lengthening from the left hip to the hand.

❸ Place the right hand on the ground behind to keep the body forward and straight.

❹ Exhale and wrap the left elbow back around the front of the right knee. Exhale, take the right arm behind and catch the left hand (with a belt if needed). Hold; repeat to the left.

(SAGE TWIST II)

Keep the breath flowing slowly and easily, using it carefully to make space: This may feel difficult once the body has turned.

Start the twist from the base of the spine and lengthen the body up and around with the exhalation.

As the armpit nears the bent knee, do not force the torso to turn: This may strain muscles between the ribs.

Take the arm around the front of the knee. This may be difficult for those with a long back and shorter legs; take time to ground the sitting bones before turning.

FOLLOW WITH:
upavistha konasana
OPEN ANGLE, PAGES 82–83

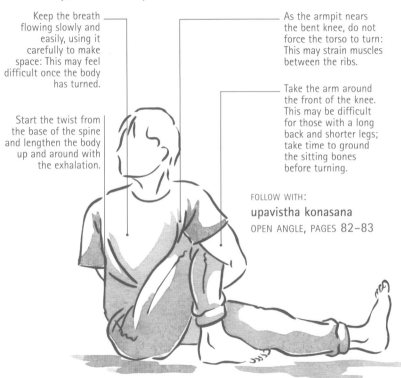

[225]

pranayama

(KHUMBHAKA–RETENTION BREATH)

Slow, calm breathing is learned using this technique, which combines a longer pause at the top of the inhalation with different lengths of inhalation and exhalation. The breath stops without tension in a moment of concentrated stillness and clarity. It is important to adopt a well-grounded sitting pose: Within the pause, the hips relax their weight down, allowing the backbone to lengthen upward. Keep the shoulders relaxed and the face calm throughout.

❶ Sitting straight and easy, start with Ujjayi breathing *(see page 25)*, move on to Kapalabhati *(see pages 123–24)*, then return to the Ujjayi breath.

❷ To start Khumbhaka, inhale to the count of 5 and exhale to the count of 10. When used to this, move on.

❸ Inhale to a count of 4, pause for 4, exhale for 8 (a ratio of 1:1:2). Continue for a few cycles, as comfortable, then return to Ujjayi. Work up to a ratio of 1:2:2 (inhale 4, pause 8, exhale 8), then 1:3:2 (inhale 4, pause 12, exhale 8).

relaxation

Start in Recuperation Pose I *(see page 26)*, then lengthen into Savasana *(see page 27)*. Notice the flow of breath never ending, meandering like a river but always progressing, and the tangible air around you: It, too, has currents. In the cocoon of relaxation let the mind observe while the body settles until the rhythm of breathing is part of the body and the mind calms, observing less, content just to be with the rhythm of the body.

1 Relax the face and jaw, back of the neck long, shoulders quiet. Feel the supportive ground and the body against it.

2 Let the outward breath pull downward and the front ribs soften, smoothing out angles and corners.

3 Feel the incoming breath expand the body with renewing and purifying air. Be aware of a simplicity in the rhythm of the breath and a center of immense beauty and quietness.

4 After five cycles of conscious breathing, open the eyes, roll to one side, and get up slowly.

the story of yoga

In the early 16th century, Babar of Kabul (a descendant of Genghis Khan) invaded India, and by 1530 had established another Islamic state that became the Mogul Empire. Its influence was to be felt throughout the sub-continent. The greatest of the Moguls was Akbar, whose religious tolerance allowed the continuance of Hindu traditions and facilitated the synthesis of Hinduism and Islam within the Sikh religion. Islamic architecture flourished alongside great poets, historians, and scholars.

Throughout these times, further literature on yoga was compiled. Yoga was, as always, part of Indian life. Gurus taught their students on a one-to-one basis, and, in turn, some of these students became teachers, with the handing down of knowledge a continuing tradition. In local communities, yogis who were particularly resonant were nurtured, and some were discovered and became famous throughout India. Lineages from this form of yoga-teaching dated back to early history and formed many different paths.

The crumbling of the Mogul Empire from the 17th century on made way for British colonial rule, which, by the mid-19th century, existed in almost all of India. The British did not integrate culturally like other invaders, but established a bureaucracy and educational system that insisted Indians learn English.

Indian thinkers soon became aware of the western world's interest in their spiritual traditions, and began to take their learning abroad. Among the first of such pioneers was Ramakrishna (1836–86), whose disciple Vivekananda (1863–1902) was an English-speaking undergraduate when he met his teacher. After Ramakrishna's death, Vivekananda, an Advaita Vedantist and jnana—studying and knowledge—yogi, left for America via China and Japan, to take part in the "Parliament of Religions" in Chicago in 1893. After four years, he returned to India and reorganized a small community of renunciants. From these roots, Ramakrishna Vedanta centers were established in India and the west, and Vivekananda began a trend for yoga in the west that continues today.

Perhaps the Indian who most influenced the west was Mohandas Karamchand Gandhi (1869–1948), born in Gujurat, the son of a government minister. His life spanned the end of British rule in India and, throughout it, he worked for modern India's independence, his philosophy influenced not only by the Jains of his local province, but by the teachings of the Bhagavad Gita. For his pacifism, idealism, and humble but persistent patriotism, Gandhi was known as Mahatma (Great Soul).

month 12

This is the last month of the yoga year, which has established clear, strong foundations for many years of rewarding study. The year has come full circle; we reflect on what we have learned and look ahead to how yoga can continue to be part of daily life.

The poses you have learned have not only stretched the body, in all senses, but stilled the mind, and so month 12 finally offers the full Lotus Pose, of special significance in yoga for breathing and meditation. The theme of the month is the quietness and stillness needed to allow the lotus to blossom, and breathwork presents the universal sound "aum."

key postures:

warming up (SUPTA PADMASANA, MATSYASANA)

eka pada rajakapotasana III (ONE LEGGED PIGEON POSE III)

ardha padmottanasana (STANDING HALF LOTUS)

ardha padma sarvangasana (SHOULDER STAND IN HALF LOTUS)

parivrtta ardha padmasana (SEATED HALF LOTUS TWIST)

padmasana (LOTUS POSE)

pranayama (AUM—VIBRATION BREATHING)

quietness and stillness

"Yoga is the stilling of the restlessness of the mind." *(Yoga Sutras)*
Asanas, or postures, prepare the body for pranayama, breathing, by
making it more flexible, toning the body so that all its systems are
working at their optimum. Such freedom from physical distraction
allows pranayama to focus purely on the breath. Pranayama, too,
affects the body, but in a more subtle way than asanas, with a finer
tuning that is interwoven with calming and quieting the mind.

This meditative state can be experienced anywhere. It is like
watching a bird in flight and being completely absorbed, not thinking
about the bird but being with it, and leaving behind other busy,
fragmented, and fleeting thoughts. In entering this state, the brain
relaxes, allowing deeper processes, intuition, or perception to surface.

The understanding that postures and breathing offer transmits
to your everyday life, work, and creativity, and the self-awareness
engendered protects you when entering different mental states.

At the core of every yoga pose there is a quietness that derives
from the combined working of the body with the mind. Within
pranayama, that quietness becomes stillness, and in the stillness
you will experience wholeness of mind, body, and spirit.

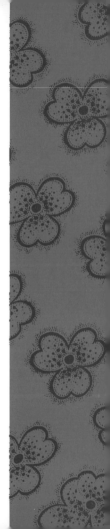

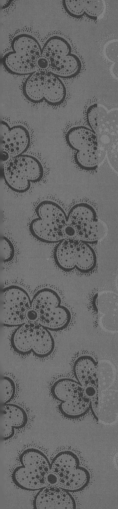

warming up

To prepare for Supta Padmasana *(see below)*, you need to warm the hips well. Start in Recuperation Pose II (page 33) and follow with the supine leg stretches on pages 34–35, then move on to Supta Gomukhasana (Cow Legs, page 111), Bhairasana (Half Yoga Sleeping Pose, page 197), and Supta Ardha Padmasana (Lying Down Half Lotus, page 133) before attempting the poses on pages 234-35.

supta padmasana (LYING DOWN LOTUS)

The supine lotus pose gives a feeling of positivity. It helps to center the body and stretches the spine away from the pelvis. In the lotus poses you must rotate the hip to enable the legs to be folded in without straining the knees. To force the pose would be to damage the body. If, at any point, you feel pain in the knee, stop and continue with other supine poses until the hips rotate more easily.

If, to begin with, the knees don't drop to the ground, place cushions beneath them and rest quietly in the pose.

supta padmasana

❶ Lying on your back, fold the right leg into half lotus *(see page 133)*, drawing it into the fold of the left leg.

❷ Draw the left knee in, turning the lower leg to hold the foot with the left hand behind the ankle, right hand behind the toes. Breathe quietly, letting the hips relax.

❸ Exhale, draw the foot over the right leg and place it in the fold of the right hip. Both knees point upward.

matsyasana (FISH POSE)

❶ From step 3, above, exhale and draw the knees in toward the body. With knees in, exhale, letting the tail-bone lengthen away and the muscles on the outside of the hips relax.

❷ Breathing out to the back of the waist, let the knees drop back and down toward the ground. Repeat all the steps on this page with legs crossed the other way.

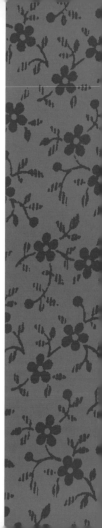

(FISH POSE)

FOLLOW WITH:

balasana CHILD POSE, PAGES 20-21

bhujangasana COBRA POSE, PAGES 112-13

eka pada rajakapotasana I
ONE LEGGED PIGEON POSE I, PAGES 54-55

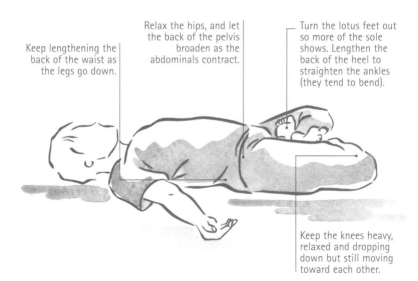

Keep lengthening the back of the waist as the legs go down.

Relax the hips, and let the back of the pelvis broaden as the abdominals contract.

Turn the lotus feet out so more of the sole shows. Lengthen the back of the heel to straighten the ankles (they tend to bend).

Keep the knees heavy, relaxed and dropping down but still moving toward each other.

eka pada rajakapotasana

(ONE LEGGED PIGEON POSE III)

This is the most advanced version of the One Legged Dove poses; even if you can't catch your foot, it's exhilarating to try and good for opening the upper back. To begin, loop a long belt around the foot, and hold it with the hands over the head. The release of the arms is similar to and helpful for Urdhva Dhanurasana (Wheel Pose, pages 202–205).

❶ Start in Eka Pada Rajakapotasana Stage I *(see pages 54-55)*, with the right leg folded under.

❷ Exhale; bringing the hands back, come up into Bhujang-asana (Cobra Pose, pages 112–13), straightening the arms, long in the back of the waist, and relaxing the hips down.

❸ When upright, bend the left leg up and, with the left hand, loop the belt around the foot, steadying yourself with the right hand.

❹ As the base settles, take the right arm over to catch the belt. Breathe, developing the pose; repeat on the right.

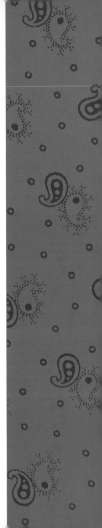

If the hands and foot are close, catch the toes while continuing to lengthen the back of the waist.

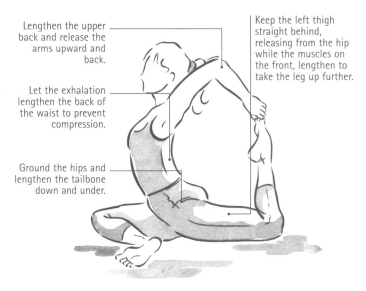

Lengthen the upper back and release the arms upward and back.

Let the exhalation lengthen the back of the waist to prevent compression.

Ground the hips and lengthen the tailbone down and under.

Keep the left thigh straight behind, releasing from the hip while the muscles on the front, lengthen to take the leg up further.

FOLLOW WITH:
pindasana AND **adho mukha svanasana sequence** CHILD POSE AND DOWNWARD FACING DOG, PAGE 23

ardha padmottanasana

(STANDING HALF LOTUS)

Before practicing this new version of lotus, revise
Tadasana (Mountain Pose, pages 14–15), Vrkasana (Tree
Pose, pages 38–39), and Utthita Hasta Padangusthasana
(Standing Hand-to-Toe, pages 116–17).

❶ From Tadasana (*see above*), take the weight onto the
right leg.

❷ Bend the left knee and take the left foot, left hand
behind the ankle, right hand behind the toes, and draw it
into half-lotus up against the thigh of the right leg.

❸ Release the left hand and take it around the back of
the waist, palm outward, to rest inside the elbow of the
right arm holding the foot.

❹ Straighten yourself by breathing out to the arm
behind, dropping the weight down the straight leg, and
lengthening upward. If the foot stays in place, take both
arms up. Come down and repeat on the other side.

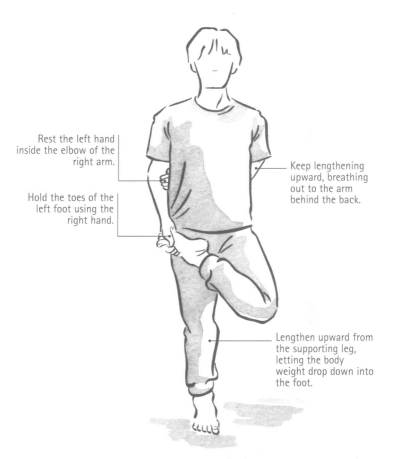

Rest the left hand inside the elbow of the right arm.

Hold the toes of the left foot using the right hand.

Keep lengthening upward, breathing out to the arm behind the back.

Lengthen upward from the supporting leg, letting the body weight drop down into the foot.

FOLLOW WITH:

uttanasana STANDING FORWARD BEND, PAGE 19

trikonasana TRIANGLE POSE, PAGES 71–75 AND **parivrtta trikonasana** TWISTING TRIANGLE, PAGES 100–101

prasarita padottanasana STANDING WIDE FORWARD BEND, PAGES 42–43

salamba sirasana HEADSTAND AND THREE POINT HEADSTAND, PAGES 178–83

sarvangasana SHOULDER STAND, PAGES 158–62 AND 184–85

ardha padma sarvangasana

(SHOULDER STAND IN HALF LOTUS)

Inverting Half Lotus (Ardha Padmottanasana, pages 238–39) makes it easier, as the hips are looser, with no weight to bear. Boost the rotation in the hip by taking the legs apart before folding the leg in.

1 From Sarvangasana *(see above)*, exhale and lengthen the torso up to the feet. Exhale and fold the right leg down, placing the side of the foot on the left thigh, sole outward.

2 To take the foot nearer the groin, bend the left knee down and wriggle the foot closer, the side strong against the thigh. Hold, then repeat on the other side.

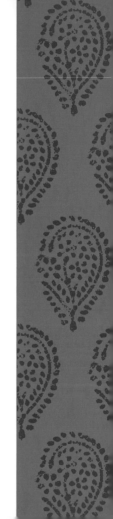

(SHOULDER STAND IN HALF LOTUS)

Press the side of the foot against the thigh and take the knee back to make the thigh vertical. Open the lotus foot outward, knee back.

Lengthen the torso on the exhalation, extending the long leg to the heel.

Drop the elbows, firm against the ground. Take the hands further up the back, toward the shoulders. Keep the hands and wrists flat against the back, to either side of the spine, fingers pointing toward the pelvis.

FOLLOW WITH:

halasana PLOW POSE, PAGES 163–65

jatara parivartanasana II SUPINE TWIST II, PAGES 78–79

ardha padma paschimottanasana SEATED HALF LOTUS FORWARD BEND, PAGES 186–187

Keep the shoulders quiet, the neck long.

parivrtta ardha padmasana

(SEATED HALF LOTUS TWIST)

This twist warms the hips and prepares for full lotus, lengthening the thigh muscles and bringing the knee to the center. Since it is better to have good knees and no lotus, if you feel strain in the knee, perform the pose as in Parivrtta Janu Shirshasana (Twisting Head-to-Knee, pages 58–59), leaving the foot on the ground.

1 Sit with the right leg straight and bend the left leg. Take the left foot with the left hand behind the ankle, right hand behind the toes, and draw it up the right thigh as high as possible without strain.

2 Exhale, relaxing the hips, feeling the sitting bones, and lengthening upward.

3 Exhale and turn to the left.

4 Exhale and take the left arm around the back of the waist, point the toes of the lotus foot, and, if within reach, catch hold of them. Repeat on the other side.

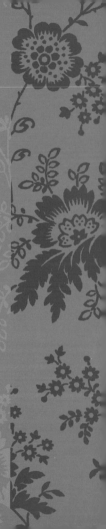

The thigh of the lotus leg comes further into the center as the body turns, and the lotus leg relaxes.

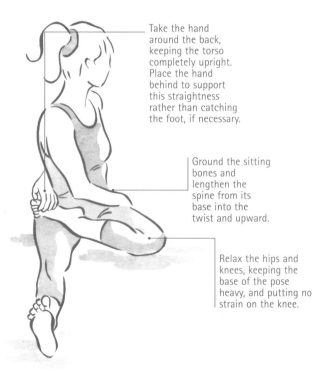

Take the hand around the back, keeping the torso completely upright. Place the hand behind to support this straightness rather than catching the foot, if necessary.

Ground the sitting bones and lengthen the spine from its base into the twist and upward.

Relax the hips and knees, keeping the base of the pose heavy, and putting no strain on the knee.

padmasana

(LOTUS POSE)

Lotus is stable because the feet anchor the thighs while the sitting bones are earthed to the floor. From this base the spine releases up, freeing the breath and making the pose ideal for breathing and meditation. It takes time to feel these effects; to begin, don't hold the pose for long. For an easier alternative, ground the base sitting cross-legged or in Ardha Padmasana (Seated Half Lotus, page 122).

❶ Start in Seated Half Lotus *(see above)*, left foot folded onto the right thigh.

❷ Bend the right leg and draw the foot in, protecting the ankle with the left hand behind the toes, the right hand behind the ankle and foot.

❸ Draw the right leg over the left and place the foot near the groin of the left thigh.

❹ Exhale and ground the sitting bones, lengthening the spine. Breathe for several cycles; repeat on the other side.

From the stable base in the sitting bones, the spine releases upward and finds its balance with the breath. The crown of the head lengthens upward with the exhalation. The shoulders are relaxed, and the back of the neck is long.

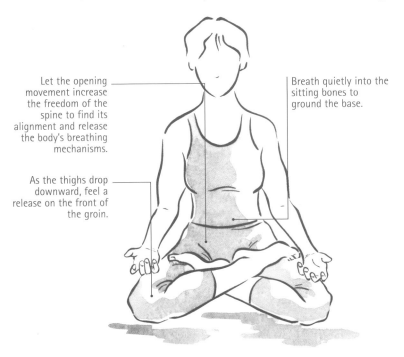

Let the opening movement increase the freedom of the spine to find its alignment and release the body's breathing mechanisms.

Breath quietly into the sitting bones to ground the base.

As the thighs drop downward, feel a release on the front of the groin.

pranayama

(AUM—VIBRATION BREATHING)

The final aim of pranayama is silence and concentration.
Vibration breaths center concentration within the body,
and by opposing silence with sound, make the silence
more complete when it returns. "Aum" is one of the oldest
sounds used for prayer and meditation, in mythology
thought to be the sound that preceded the forming of the
universe. Its vowels "a" ("aah") and "u" ("oo") stretch the
facial muscles and work the jaw, while the "mmm" forms
the vibration on the exhalation.

❶ Sitting straight, start Ujjayi breathing (see page 25),
add Kapalabhati (see pages 123–24), and return to Ujjayi.

❷ Let in an inhalation. At the top of the in-breath, with
no pause and with the out-breath, open the mouth to form
the sounds "a" and "oo", and close the lips on "mmmm,"
letting the hum move down the body with the out-breath.

❸ Inhale; repeat the "aum" on the exhalation. Continue
for several cycles before returning to Ujjayi breathing.

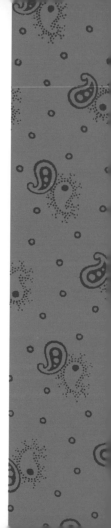

relaxation

Start in Recuperation Pose I *(see page 26)*, then lengthen into Savasana *(see page 27)*. Let the body's undulations even out on the ground. Relax the hips, back of the waist long, legs heavy, pelvis broad and stable. Feel the breath like a sigh, shoulders and arms relaxed. As the mind quietens, do nothing but be absolutely in contact with the breath. The mind is alert, in unison with the whole of you. There is no separation, only a joining of body and mind, with the security of the ground beneath forming the contact with reality.

1 Broaden the forehead, eyes closed and looking down.

2 Sense the in-breath cool on the upper lip, the out-breath warm. The ears widen behind the head: Hear distant sounds.

3 Let the inhalation travel in freely, and follow the out-breath unfolding down the whole inside of the spine.

4 After five cycles of breath, open the eyes. Enjoy the newness of sight. Roll to one side, stretch to regain contact with the body; get up slowly.

the story of yoga

During the 20th century, yoga was increasingly embraced by the west. Gurus of every description arrived from India, and many became famous or infamous (the history of yoga in India has seen many disagreements, strange sects and cults have always abounded, and gurus are, after all, only human). Some of these individuals brought with them yoga techniques, traditions, and ways of thinking that have greatly enriched the story of yoga and increased its accessibility in the west.

The Maharishi Mahesh Yogi, born in Mahesh Varma in 1917, founded Transcendental Meditation. He taught the liberation of human consciousness, and his secular style was in keeping with the trends of the 1960s toward personal self-development and freedom. Pop stars, such as The Beatles, visited the Maharishi, creating a new level of publicity that increased the appeal of Indian spirituality in the west.

The majority of yoga taught in the west today is a form of Hatha yoga that focuses on practicing asanas and pranayama to achieve better health and well-being. Yet yoga is not a purely Indian art. Many other countries have deep-rooted yoga traditions, both secular and religious, including those derived from the different forms of Buddhism, from Sufism, and from Chinese belief systems. There is yoga of health, yoga of energy, and yoga of psychic mysteries, and in major cities throughout the west, one can study every variety of yoga technique.

Coming out of the ancient Indian tradition of teaching yoga on a one-to-one basis, single gurus who preached their own form of yoga to a large audience were much in evidence in the 20th century. Alongside these teachers, schools of yoga developed to disseminate ideas and philosophies developed from varied sources. Yoga is not a static phenomenon, and, throughout the world, teachers are constantly developing new styles of yoga adapted to suit the needs of their own culture and the way of life of their specific audience.

This is the way yoga will develop in the 21st century, and it is a testimony to the readily adaptive quality of the system: Yoga has withstood 4,000 years of development, and, whatever our reasons for taking it up, perhaps, in our own yoga practice, we are not so different to the Harappan householder sitting down on a sunny morning to contemplate her gods, or the Vedic-Aryan warrior, pausing in his migration to observe the wonders of nature.

Yoga, through clear introspection, provides answers to the questions: Who am I? and Where am I going? There is as much need within the materialism of the west for this form of spirituality as there has ever been.

the backbone

The spine is a series of bony segments, vertebrae, with disks of cartilage between that act as shock absorbers. The spinal cord, which runs toward the back of the spine and is protected by the vertebrae, contains the main nerves that send messages to and from the brain. These nerves control all the body's systems, including the muscular, circulatory, digestive, and endocrine systems, making the health of the spine integral to the health of the body.

In a standing position, the backbone curves like a serpentine to support the different loads of the three main masses of the body-the head, chest, and pelvis. Although these natural curves withstand the force of gravity, the intervertebral discs suffer from compression. You can see this by noticing how, after sleeping at night, the body is slightly taller in the morning. The vertebrae, along with other joints in the body, also become distorted through lifestyle, stress, and trauma.

Yoga asanas help to keep the joints in the body mobile. They focus on the backbone since all movement is connected to it, and breathing is part of that movement. Asanas also use gravity to help the alignment of the body, and to lessen the strain on joints while performing the poses.

THE SKELETON

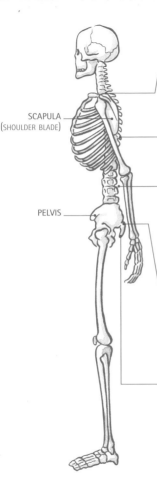

SCAPULA
(SHOULDER BLADE)

PELVIS

CERVICAL VERTEBRAE The concave curve of these seven small vertebrae balances the weight of the head. Lengthening the back of the neck and head brings the chin level, to balance the head more easily.

THORACIC VERTEBRAE The weight of the chest and lungs pulls the thoracic spine forward. The ribs, connected to the thoracic, are moved by breathing, which in turn moves the spine. By lengthening the thoracic spine with the exhalation, weight from the chest is dispersed upward and downward.

LUMBAR VERTEBRAE The inner curve of the lumbar spine balances the upper body with the lower, allowing free movement. Letting the lower back drop more vertically helps correct the lumbar into its natural curve and frees it to become more mobile.

SACRUM The sacrum slots into the back of the pelvis and transfers weight from the upper body through the hips to the legs and ground. The sacrum takes a lot of pressure, and widening the back of the pelvis helps it to pinch less tightly into its slot.

COCCYX The tailbone curls down and under, between the sitting bones, the narrow bones at the bottom of the pelvic girdle.

the lungs

Breathing is an involuntary reflex—we can hold the breath, but it's impossible to stop it completely. Although we don't have to learn to breathe, many of us suffer imbalances in the way we breathe: Breathing shallowly uses only part of the lungs; bad posture adversely affects the freedom of the chest cavity; and emotions from depression to shock can contract and compress the chest, hindering effective breathing.

The diaphragm is the main operator in the mechanics of breathing, rhythmically contracting and relaxing. It contracts and flattens with the inhalation, effortlessly drawing air into the lungs, then relaxes back and up on the exhalation. As the exhalation is longer than the inhalation, the diaphragm spends more time resting, enabling it to maintain its constant function, and boosting the oxygenating capacity of the lungs. Other muscles help the exhalation and connect it with movement. If the abdominal muscles contract, the curve in the lower back lengthens, relaxing the spinal muscles along with the diaphragm. This allows the backbone to extend while the pelvis, dropping away from the waist, frees the legs.

Breathing effectively improves the oxygenation and detoxification of the body. Yoga is of immense benefit in establishing correct breathing patterns, which help extend and realign the spine.

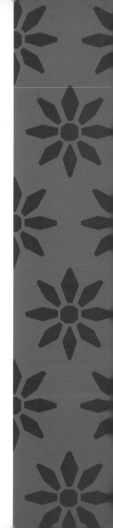

THE LUNGS, DIAPHRAGM, AND MOVEMENT

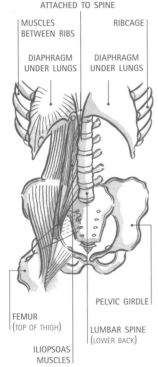

STEM OF DIAPHRAGM
ATTACHED TO SPINE

MUSCLES
BETWEEN RIBS

RIBCAGE

DIAPHRAGM
UNDER LUNGS

DIAPHRAGM
UNDER LUNGS

PELVIC GIRDLE

FEMUR
(TOP OF THIGH)

LUMBAR SPINE
(LOWER BACK)

ILIOPSOAS
MUSCLES

LUNGS Air travels down the windpipe and bronchial passages into the lungs, where oxygen is absorbed into the bloodstream and carried to the heart to be pumped around the body. Carbon dioxide is carried back to the lungs and expelled with the exhalation.

DIAPHRAGM The mushroom-shaped diaphragm sits attached to and inside the lower ribs beneath the lungs, separating the chest cavity from the abdomen. It contracts and flattens with the inhalation. As the chest cavity lengthens, the lungs expand, forming a vacuum. To equalize pressure, air is drawn in, and the diaphragm relaxes back and up, shortening the chest cavity and pressing down on the lungs, causing pressure to increase and air to be expelled.

LUMBAR SPINE The stem of the diaphragm attaches to the lumbar spine and meets the iliopsoas muscles running down the inside of the spine through the pelvis to the tops of the legs.

ILIOPSOAS MUSCLES These spinal muscles integrate upper and lower body movements, and affect the curve in the lower back by tilting the pelvis. When the abdominal muscles contract with the out-breath, they support the spine while the diaphragm and iliopsoas muscles relax.

how to practice and form your routines

Daily practice is best but sometimes this is impossible. If you find it hard to practice, do not let it sabotage your desire to do yoga. Practice when you can and each time this will help you to want to practice more. Find a time to practice that is suitable for you. There are no rules and some prefer the morning, others prefer the evening.

For the first three months, practice for 20 minutes: 10 minutes for the poses, 5 for breathing (pranayama) and 5 for relaxation. In the second quarter these times will increase.

To do the poses in the third and fourth quarters, you will need to be practicing more regularly and for longer (45 minutes to 1 hour). It is better to practice for shorter times regularly rather than a long time in one session sporadically.

When you have become used to the routines in *The Yoga Year*, you will be able to form your own routines. The routines in this book have started with lying down poses, followed by kneeling, standing, inverted, sitting, pranayama and relaxation. A balanced approach includes at least two or three of these sections though the order can vary. Always end with relaxation.

1 Start with easier poses before working up to harder ones. In between poses there is rest, or the counterbalance of one pose with another. Backbends are followed by forward bends or twists. Twists can be done at any point of the practice but always do them on each side.

2 With the inverted poses, make sure you have thoroughly warmed up before doing them. Follow head balance with shoulder balance and shoulder balance with the supine twist or dog.

3 Sitting poses at the end prepare you for sitting in pranayama. It is best to end the routine on a symmetrical pose like one of the forward bends. Give yourself 5 minutes for breathing (pranayama) and 5 or 10 minutes for relaxation.

4 Eventually you may find that you would like a teacher to check your symmetry and take you further forward. There may be a local class that you can attend or a weekend course that you can travel to. There are many different sorts of yoga that are taught and therefore try different approaches until you find one that suits you. *The Yoga Year* will then remain as a guide and encouragement to your routines.

section IV index